GERIATRICS

GERIATRICS

Carol Leth Stone

Health and Medical Issues Today

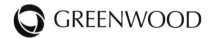

AN IMPRINT OF ABC-CLIO, LLC
Santa Barbara, California • Denver, Colorado • Oxford, England

Library of Congress Cataloging-in-Publication Data

Stone, Carol Leth.
    Geriatrics / Carol Leth Stone.
        p. ; cm. — (Health and medical issues today)
    Includes bibliographical references and index.
    ISBN 978-0-313-37618-4 (hard copy : alk. paper) — ISBN 978-0-313-37619-1
(eISBN)   1. Geriatrics   2. Aging.   I. Title.   II. Series: Health and medical issues today.
    [DNLM: 1. Geriatrics.   2. Aged—physiology.   3. Aged—psychology.
    4. Aging—physiology.   WT 100]
    RC952.S78   2011
    618.97—dc22   2011002270

ISBN: 978-0-313-37618-4
EISBN: 978-0-313-37619-1

15 14 13 12 11   1 2 3 4 5

This book is also available on the World Wide Web as an eBook.
Visit www.abc-clio.com for details.

Greenwood
An Imprint of ABC-CLIO, LLC

ABC-CLIO, LLC
130 Cremona Drive, P.O. Box 1911
Santa Barbara, California 93116-1911

This book is printed on acid-free paper ∞

Manufactured in the United States of America

In memory of Harold J. Stone
Husband and friend for 32 years

CONTENTS

SERIES FOREWORD

Every day, the public is bombarded with information on developments in medicine and health care. Whether the focus is on the latest techniques in treatments or research or concerns over public health threats, this information directly impacts the lives of people more than almost any other issue. Although there are many sources for understanding these topics—from Web sites and blogs to newspapers and magazines—students and ordinary citizens often need one resource that makes sense of the complex health and medical issues affecting their daily lives.

The *Health and Medical Issues Today* series provides just such a one-stop resource for obtaining a solid overview of the most controversial areas of health care today. Each volume addresses one topic and provides a balanced summary of what is known. These volumes provide an excellent first step for students and laypeople interested in understanding how health care works in our society today.

Each volume is broken into several sections to provide readers and researchers with easy access to the information they need:

- Part I provides overview chapters on background information—including chapters on such areas as the historical, scientific, medical, social, and legal issues involved—that a citizen needs to intelligently understand the topic.
- Part II provides capsule examinations of the most heated contemporary issues and debates and analyzes in a balanced manner the viewpoints held by various advocates in the debates.

- Part III provides a selection of reference material, such as annotated primary source documents, a timeline of important events, and a directory of organizations that serve as the best next step in learning about the topic at hand.

The *Health and Medical Issues Today* series strives to provide readers with all the information needed to begin making sense of some of the most important debates going on in the world today. The series includes volumes on such topics as stem-cell research, obesity, gene therapy, alternative medicine, organ transplantation, mental health, and more.

PREFACE

Concern about medicine and services for the elderly has grown in recent years, along with the increase in life expectancy in developed countries. As a result, the medical specialty known as geriatrics has become ever more important. In addition, researchers are carrying out studies of the elderly in the science called gerontology.

Physicians and scientists may seem to be the main actors in geriatric care and studies, but the elderly need to take responsibility for themselves in some matters and to seek reliable help for others. In a technological era when even many of the very old use the World Wide Web and communicate with e-mail and texting, it is possible to educate oneself to a large extent and to take charge of health and other issues.

Although we may avoid thinking about age-related issues when we are young, at some point—such as when we are invited to join the American Association of Retired Persons (AARP) at age 50—we all begin to do so. In my own case, years of caregiving and then becoming a widow in my mid-60s greatly focused my attention on issues of aging. Besides that, during the writing of this book, my mother died at the age of 101 years. I had been intimately involved in every aspect of her care for several years.

Dealing with aging can be bewildering, for ourselves or on behalf of others. We need to work with physicians to ensure good medical care; to be aware of financial and legal traps; to assert ourselves when younger people condescend to us; and to handle a myriad of other large and small issues. It is my hope that this reference will be of some help to those who need it—to the elderly and their health care providers.

ACKNOWLEDGMENTS

Much of this book was written at the Marshall Community Health Library in Placerville, California. The librarians, especially Community Health Librarian Alison Clement, helped greatly with my research. I am extremely grateful to them and to the donors who support this important community resource. Kathy Hanley, PT, at the Elders Inn in Alameda, California, gave me valuable information relating to physical therapy for elderly people. Vicki Ludwig, chair of the El Dorado County Commission on Aging, helped me find material on societal issues.

Helpful friends and relatives have contributed much, also. My late mother, Isabelle Beall, and I talked about many geriatric issues over the years, as we both dealt with the problems and rewards of getting older. John and Anna Owens, Joani Blank, and Lorraine Peterson provided valuable suggestions and advice on various portions of the rough draft. Ruth Levitan allowed me to include her moving poem about aging, "Indian Summer." Most of all, my beloved companion Thane Puissegur helped me throughout the long writing process, listening to my complaints, making suggestions for additions, and helping me revise rough drafts.

Having spent many years as an editor, I am extremely aware of the contributions good editors make. I greatly appreciate the comments and assistance of both Michael Nobel, ABC-CLIO senior acquisitions editor, and Caryl Boyer, copyeditor. In addition, Diane Worden did her usual thorough job on the index.

PART I

Overview

The Growing
Geriatric Population

In the year 1900, life expectancy at birth in the United States averaged only 47 years; by the end of the century, it had increased to more than 75 years (Barker, 1998). Although the increase can be attributed mainly to lowered infant mortality, the average life expectancy for those who have reached age 65 has also grown—from 76 years in 1900 to 81 years today for men, and even more for women. This is already leading to a rise in the over-85 group, which will grow even more as more of the baby boomers become elderly. In 1980, only about 1 in 100 Americans was older than 85; by 2050, it is projected that more than 1 in 25 will be that old. In 1990, there were 3.25 million persons aged 85 or more, representing 10% of those over 65; in 2010, there are 5.8 million, or 14% of those over 65. About 60% of the over-85 are women, who tend to be poorer than men because they are likely to have worked for smaller salaries or for shorter periods under Social Security. All of this obviously creates a great economic burden for the country.

Current government projections about the burgeoning population of elderly people and the resulting negative effects on society and the economy are pessimistic, but the actual situation may become even worse. In a recent article (Olshansky et al., 2009), it is argued that future life expectancy may increase more than predicted. According to the Social Security Administration's forecasts, in 2050, life expectancy at birth will rise to 80.0 years for men and 83.4 years for women. (The corresponding figures for Census

Bureau predictions are 80.9 and 85.3.) According to the Olshansky et al. report, death rates may be reduced by 2050 because of medical progress against major fatal diseases, which would bring about an even higher life expectancy of 83.2 years for men and 89.2 years for women. Although that may be a positive effect from individuals' point of view, it will cause financial and other difficulties for society. As just one effect, by 2050, the cumulative costs for Medicare and Social Security may rise to $8.3 trillion.

On the other hand, the report indicates that there also may be some gains. As people live longer, they may have access to better medical care and have more years of leisure. Businesses will benefit if workers are more experienced.

It might be expected, of course, that, as the elderly population increases, the field of medicine known as geriatrics will increase as well.

CHAPTER 1

Geriatrics as a Medical Specialty

Like much of Western medicine, geriatrics dates back at least as far as Hippocrates, the "father of medicine," who lived to be about 90 years old himself. (He is believed to have been born ca. 460 B.C.E., and to have died ca. 370 B.C.E.) Hippocrates observed that "Old men suffer from difficulty of breathing, catarrh accompanied by coughing, strangury [straining to urinate], difficulty of micturition, pains at the joints, kidney disease, dizziness, apoplexy, cachexia [physical wasting], pruritus of the whole body, sleeplessness, watery discharge from the bowels, eyes and nostrils, dullness of sight, cataract, hardness of hearing" (quoted in Howell, 1986). Hippocrates' definition of "elderly" was the ages between 49 and 57; anyone over 57 was defined as "old."

Hippocrates recognized stroke as sudden paralysis and called it apoplexy. However, the physical basis of stroke was not recognized until the 17th century: In 1620, the Swiss physician Jacob Webfer performed autopsies on stroke victims and discovered that bleeding into their brains had occurred. In addition, Webfer studied the carotid and vertebral arteries and realized that when they are blocked, too little blood reaches the brain tissue. The result is a stroke (National Institute of Neurological Disorders and Stroke, 2010a).

Avicenna, an Arab scholar in the 10th century, was a major figure in the history of medicine who tried to combine Galen's and Aristotle's philosophy with Arabic knowledge (Howell, 1987). In his *Canon of Medicine*, Avicenna paid special attention to the elderly, thus becoming the precursor of modern geriatricians. His Regimen of Old Age emphasized the importance of sleep; Avicenna said that the elderly need more sleep than younger people do.

Much like the physicians of today, Avicenna encouraged the elderly to exercise but not to do so strenuously. He favored horse riding and walking as the best forms of exercise for the elderly.

In the Middle Ages, bleeding was commonly used as a draconian cure for various disorders. However, it was considered too rigorous for elderly patients, and so they were not subjected to it (Martin, 2008). Also, according to Martin's study of works by four medieval surgeons, surgery was not routinely performed on anyone over 70. In the centuries before anesthetics, the pain of surgery would have been excruciating for anyone, especially a frail, aged person.

Surgery that might have cured some elderly patients was impossible for centuries because it was so painful and stressful that patients could not survive the surgery. That all changed in the early 19th century, when Crawford Williamson Long, a U.S. physician, began the use of ether to anesthetize surgical patients. When other doctors complained that he was using a dangerous new poison on his patients, Long gave up any quest for recognition (Lehrer, 1979). The credit is usually given instead to a dentist, William Morton, who used ether for very painful dental procedures in the 1840s. Later, chloroform and other anesthetics became more common. By making painless surgery possible, anesthetics surely saved countless lives of elderly patients.

For many elderly patients, weakened hearts cannot pump blood throughout the body, and so fluid accumulates. Today, we call the condition cardiac edema; in earlier times, it was called dropsy. Among other victims, the great lexicographer Samuel Johnson died painfully of dropsy in 1784.

Folk medicines had long been used for dropsy. Powdered toad skins and plant sources of glycosides were used in concoctions that benefited many sufferers (Lehrer, 1979). Digitalis, the primary medicine even today for treating weakened heart muscles, was for centuries obtained from the purple foxglove plant, *Digitalis purpurea*. It is still of major importance for those with heart disease, a large portion of whom are elderly. In the late 18th century, William Withering, an English physician, discovered that medicines containing digitalis could cure patients with heart failure. This was a major advancement in geriatrics.

Although the word *geriatrics* was coined in 1909 by a U.S. physician, Ignatz Nascher, the field did not receive the support in the United States that it did in England (Evans, 1997). In particular, Marjory Warren took a special interest in medicine for the elderly. Today Warren is considered a heroine who revolutionized medical care for the elderly (Evans, 1997).

After World War II, the United Kingdom established the National Health Service, which has greatly benefited the elderly. At the same time,

---

MARJORY WARREN (1897–1960)

In 19th-century England, the elderly poor were often sent to work-houses. As Charles Dickens had made famous, workhouses were scarcely fit for habitation by the young and healthy, much less the frail old. In the early 1900s, the physician Marjory Warren took on the re-sponsibility of reforming the workhouses and providing better care for the elderly. She established a system of assigning the elderly to various blocks in a public assistance institution, making it easier to treat them according to their needs (Warren, 1943). She urged the medical estab-lishment to expand the field that was later named geriatrics, to provide medical care that was especially appropriate for the old. Rather than emphasizing patients' anatomy and physiology alone, Warren used a holistic multidisciplinary approach, taking their social and physical environments into consideration as well (Matthews, 1984). At West Middlesex Hospital, she improved patients' surroundings and intro-duced rehabilitation programs. She also wrote 27 articles on geriatrics.

---

geriatrics was established as a medical specialty there, and every medi-cal school and hospital had departments of geriatrics (John A. Hartford Foundation, 2010).

Owing to the efforts of Warren and others, geriatrics has continued to be an important part of medical education and practice in the United Kingdom. It has not been without political problems, however (Evans, 1997). At first, geriatricians were appointed to spots in teaching hospitals but were denied access to private practice, which led to their being perceived as inferior to physicians in other medical specialties. During the 1970s, the government briefly considered taking resources from other branches of medicine and transferring them to geriatrics, causing resentment from the other disci-plines and a general feeling that the elderly were taking up more than their share of space and funds. When the government withdrew the proposed change, resentment died down.

Once known as the "old man's friend" because it killed many of the elderly who might otherwise die from far more painful causes, pneumo-nia became much less prevalent after penicillin was discovered and made available. Sir Alexander Fleming, a Scottish physician and researcher, in 1928 noticed a large, clear area in a culture dish overgrown with staphy-lococci. He realized that bacteria there had been killed by a mold that had contaminated the dish and that the mold must contain some antibacterial substance. Later work by Fleming and others led to the development of penicillin (Lehrer, 1979).

Today many bacteria have developed resistance to penicillin and its derivatives, such as methicillin. The bacteria *Staphylococcus aureus,* especially, now leads to many methicillin-resistant *Staphylococcus aureus* (MRSA) infections. However, the antibiotics first found by Fleming still control many infections that affect the elderly and others.

In the United States, Ignatz Leo Nascher (1863–1944) was by far the major figure in this field, writing the textbook *Geriatrics* and promoting the subject throughout his life (Achenbaum, 2004). According to Achenbaum, Nascher had little support from other physicians and in 1926 considered himself the only practicing geriatrician in the United States. However, he continued to urge the medical profession to study and treat the old, and he founded the New York Geriatrics Society. Aging was considered pathological at the time, but Nascher emphasized the physiology of aging, comparing it with the special physiology of children. He believed that there was an aversion to treating the elderly: "In the aged the repugnance aroused by the disagreeable facial aspect and the idea of economic worthlessness destroys the sympathy we bestow upon the child and instills a spirit of irritability if not positive enmity against the helplessness of the aged" (Nascher, 1916). However, interest in caring for the elderly did increase along with their proportion of the total population, and in 1942 a group of concerned physicians established the American Geriatrics Society (AGS). Lucien Stark was appointed the first president.

The AGS publishes the monthly magazine *Geriatrics* and peer-reviewed publications, including *Journal of the American Geriatrics Society, Annals of Long-term Care,* and *Clinical Geriatrics.* Its annual meetings provide a forum for researchers and clinicians to present their findings and recommendations. Originally limited to geriatricians, membership in the AGS is now open to other professional health workers who are involved with the elderly.

The work begun by Marjory Warren in England ultimately benefited the United States when Paul Beeson, who had been a professor of medicine at Oxford University, came to the United States and began urging the medical profession to expand the field of geriatrics (John A. Hartford Foundation, 2010). In 1978, Beeson led the Institute of Medicine to issue the first of a series of reports on aging. The report, titled "Aging and Medical Education," urged medical schools and teaching hospitals to make aging part of the curriculum for medical students and residents. The National Institute on Aging was begun in 1974 by the National Institutes of Health. A year later, the Veterans Health Administration (the medical division of the U.S. Department of Veterans Affairs, or the VA) set up centers to benefit veterans (Geriatric Research, Education and Clinical Care Centers). Also in 1978, the VA established two-year fellowship programs in geriatrics at some VA medical centers. The numbers of these fellowship programs later increased, growing to 93 programs in 1986. In the beginning, fellowships usually lasted two years. After a second Institute of Medicine study appeared in 1987, recommending the establishment of Centers of Excellence in geriatrics, geriatric fellowships were expanded. The John A. Hartford Foundation funded the first of these centers.

The American Boards of Family Practice and Internal Medicine established the Certificate of Added Qualifications (CAQ) in geriatric medicine in 1988. The CAQ required two years of fellowship training. The Accreditation Council for Graduate Medical Education also accredited 62 internal medicine fellowship programs and 16 family practice geriatric medicine programs. To increase the number of applicants to these programs, the two-year requirement was changed to one year in 1998 (a move that was opposed by some gerontologists). Between then and 2002, 10,207 physicians were certified in geriatric medicine.

Even today, geriatric medicine is relegated to a department of internal medicine in many universities. However, in 1982, the Mount Sinai School of Medicine established the first department of geriatrics, and medical schools in the United States have six departments of geriatrics. In addition, there is some provision for geriatrics in the structure of 105 U.S. medical schools.

Along with the expansion of geriatrics as a medical specialty, gerontology (research on aging) has grown rapidly during the past 30 years. The National Institute on Aging has received enormous government support. Other departments in the National Institutes of Health that are carrying out much research on aging are the National Heart, Lung and Blood Institute, the National Eye Institute, the National Cancer Institute, the National Institute of Musculoskeletal Disease, and the National Institute of Mental Health. Private foundations also support research on disorders that affect the elderly and on the aging process.

Despite improvements in the field's status in recent decades, there is a shortage of physicians who have been trained in geriatrics in the United States. The outlook for geriatric care today appears rather dismal, because the field is unattractive to many medical students, who are likely to emerge from medical school with large debts for their training. Medical school graduates in 2007 owed an average of $138,608 for their education (American Geriatrics Society, 2010). Of all medical specialties, geriatrics pays the least to physicians, although the training is at least as expensive as that for family medicine. Geriatricians train at least a year longer than their primary care colleagues, and yet they are compensated at a lower level. In 2006, the average annual income among geriatricians was $168,000. (For comparison, this was $2,133 less than the average annual salary of family physicians and $15,171 less than the average annual income among general internists.) Those who do choose geriatrics as a specialty are likely to have received their medical degrees outside the United States, which, for some doctors, means they will leave the country later.

How many physicians for the elderly will there be in the future? Unfortunately, the specialty of geriatrics is not growing as rapidly as the aging population is. According to the American Geriatrics Society, there are 7,590 certified geriatricians in the United States—or 1 geriatrician for every 2,500 Americans 75 or older. Bad as that is, because of the projected increase in the number of older persons, the ratio is expected to change to 1 geriatrician for every 4,254 older Americans in the year 2030. So a medical student of today who is considering specializing in geriatrics is faced with caring for a very large number of patients for a relatively small income.

Physicians who do remain in geriatrics receive less income than other physicians, in part because much of their income comes from Medicare, which tends to pay less than private insurance plans do. This imbalance is even more prevalent in mental health services. Some geriatricians and family practice physicians now refuse to accept new Medicare patients because of the low payments, but that causes a further problem: anyone over the age of 65 is unlikely *not* to be a Medicare patient.

A geriatrician has an MD degree and is board certified in family medicine or internal medicine as well as board certified in geriatrics. This qualifies him or her to give the elderly the special care they need—prescribing drugs in a manner that is appropriate for older people, working with patients and families, and cooperating with other medical team members to address a variety of problems that may be present. After earning their MDs, geriatricians complete a three-year residency program before entering a geriatric medicine fellowship program.

During their training, geriatricians become expert in the physiology of aging; illnesses common among the elderly; symptoms of illnesses that appear differently in older adults than the way they appear in younger people; the care of elderly adults in various settings, such as nursing homes and hospices; and the assessment of cognitive status and mood in the elderly. In addition to this training in caring for ill people, geriatricians have clinical training and experience in providing care for persons who are generally healthy and mainly require preventive health care. Preventive health care may be needed frequently and require much supervision by the physician.

Geriatricians' training also highlights behavioral aspects of illness, socio-economic factors, health literacy issues, and ethical and legal considerations that may affect the medical management of older patients more than that of younger people. They often work as part of a team in assessing and treating patients. Nurses, pharmacists, and physical therapists—some of whom may also have training in geriatrics—are some other health providers who may be on a patient's team.

Some geriatricians may undergo additional training to become certified as geropsychiatrists, psychiatrists who are especially attuned to the emotional needs and illnesses of the elderly. Geropsychiatrists complete a four-year residency program in psychiatry before entering a fellowship program in geriatric psychiatry. In addition, there is a growing need for geropsychologists—psychologists with educations at many levels, including doctorates, who specialize in helping elderly patients. Depending on how much education they have, some geropsychologists can prescribe medicines, much as an MD can, and others are restricted to counseling.

In April 2008, there were 7,590 board-certified geriatricians and 1,657 board-certified geriatric psychiatrists in the United States. These numbers represent a small fraction of the number of geriatric patients, and the proportion will become smaller as the elderly population increases. Only about half of the fellowship training slots are filled each year. There is currently 1 geropsychiatrist for every 11,451 patients, and, by 2030, each psychiatrist will represent 20,195 eligible patients. A possible bright spot in physicians' financial picture is that geriatricians who provide hospital-based care for the elderly and hospital-based palliative care have been in greater demand and are earning more competitive salaries in recent years.

HEALTH AND SAFETY ISSUES ASSOCIATED WITH AGING

Some diseases are found mainly in elderly people; others are found in all age groups but are more serious or must be treated differently in the elderly. In either case, individualized treatment is important.

In working with elderly patients, physicians need to use somewhat different considerations than those appropriate for younger patients. For example, a general practitioner is unlikely to examine the feet of a 30-year-old unless there is a specific problem. For 80-year-olds, though, foot examinations are highly relevant; patients may be arthritic and unable to reach down and cut their toenails, or they may have poor vision that makes it difficult for them to care for their feet. Uncut or badly trimmed nails can lead to sores and serious infections.

Like the feet, the rest of the skeleton may present disorders in elderly patients. Bone density declines with age and may lead to osteoporosis, especially in women. Thus, routine bone-density tests are needed. Many patients can benefit from increased sun exposure, which stimulates their bodies' production of vitamin D, and from calcium and vitamin D supplements.

A related problem that is more pronounced with age is strength and balance. The risk from falls is great, because so many of the elderly have osteopenia or osteoporosis and can easily break bones. A physician can assess a patient's strength and ability to balance fairly easily by observing the patient walking, standing, and sitting.

Like physical strength, mental ability is likely to decline in the elderly. Physicians need to question patients about whether they have problems with memory. Dementias of various kinds and degrees may be present. Alzheimer's disease is now among the 10 leading causes of death for older white persons but not for other racial groups. The reasons for the disparity are unclear. The increase may be due to improvements in diagnosis and reporting as well as to greater incidence of the disease. Dementia may also result from a stroke or trauma. Physicians need to be alert for signs of confusion and problems with memory and refer some patients to a neurologist for further testing.

Patients themselves may have unexpressed worries about their health that physicians may overlook. As a result, the patients suffer needlessly from treatable disorders. Incontinence, for instance, is an extremely limiting condition for many elderly; yet, they may think it is untreatable or feel embarrassed to mention it. Similarly, treatable sexual problems may be hidden by patients. Failing vision and hearing are common and may be treatable or related to other medical problems.

Some patients may need age-appropriate advice about nutrition and exercise. Having heard conflicting reports about nutrition and exercise at various times in their lives, they may feel unable to decide what they need, or they may distrust doctors who seem to "change their minds every few years." Most of the elderly can benefit from a light, conservative diet that provides vitamins and minerals, a balance of nutrients (proteins, carbohydrates, and fats), fiber, and water; special foods are seldom necessary and may be a needless expense. Similarly, they do not usually need to join a gym or try to run marathons—walking for half an hour a day provides beneficial exercise for most people and can be supplemented with more strenuous activity if desired.

Many of the elderly have problems with alcohol that may not be apparent to medical providers. A glass of red wine each day can promote health for many older people, but it should be used cautiously. Alcohol abuse or toxicity can occur when people do not realize that their tolerance for alcohol has declined or when they take medications that should not be combined with alcohol.

In general, the digestive system continues to function well into aging. When digestive problems arise, they tend to result from a poor diet, too little exercise, disease, or the effects of drugs. In many of the elderly, gums recede and teeth are lost. Although age is a contributing factor, poor oral hygiene and lack of dental care are more likely to be causes of dental problems.

In sum, the geriatrician or other physician seeing an elderly patient needs to take the whole person into account. It may be appropriate to disregard certain medical problems in the very old or to pay special attention to something that sounds trivial at first. For instance, neither geriatric physicians nor their patients need to be overly concerned about small wrinkles in the skin. But a patient who seems nervous or afraid out of proportion to the medical visit should not be ignored, because it may be an indication that the patient has dementia or is being subjected to elder abuse. Some sympathetic questions may elicit helpful information.

Causes of Death

Chronic diseases bring about most deaths among the elderly. Heart disease and cancer have led other causes of death among persons 65 years of age and older for the past two decades. Heart disease, including heart attacks and chronic ischemic heart disease, caused 35% of all deaths, and cancer caused 22% (Sahyoun et al., 2001).

Other important chronic diseases among the elderly include stroke (cerebrovascular disease), chronic obstructive pulmonary disease (COPD), diabetes, pneumonia, and influenza.

There is some variation among different groups of the elderly as to the leading causes of death. Heart disease remains the leading cause of death for most of the groups. Cancer is as common as heart disease within the youngest age group, 65 to 74 years of age, but is less important in the oldest group, ranking third among women 85 years of age and older.

For the elderly as a whole, stroke is the third leading cause of death. However, the third leading cause for white men and women aged 65 to 74 is chronic obstructive pulmonary disease, which includes chronic bronchitis, emphysema, asthma, and other chronic respiratory diseases. COPD, deaths from which are believed to be caused primarily by cigarette smoking, is the fourth or fifth cause of death for most nonwhites.

An elderly person is likely to suffer from more than one life-threatening condition at the time of death, and it is difficult in some cases for the attending physician to identify the main cause of death. Death certificates may list up to 20 diseases and conditions in addition to the underlying cause of death.

Several important renal diseases (including nephritis, nephritic syndrome, and nephrosis) have increased their tolls as causes of death among the elderly over the past 20 years. Renal diseases rank between sixth and tenth as a cause of death. They are a greater cause of death among black people than among whites.

Infectious diseases were once the major killers of the elderly, but they have been replaced by chronic conditions. Even today, however, pneumonia, influenza, and septicemia remain among the top 10 causes of death at all ages. Infectious diseases were responsible for 215,143 U.S. deaths in 2006 (Centers for Disease Control and Prevention, 2006). This role in declining health and mortality is partly hidden: some medical conditions that are preceded by infectious diseases, such as endocarditis and rheumatic heart disease, are classified as heart diseases.

Somewhat surprisingly, the combined death rate from pneumonia and influenza has increased in recent years for people of all ages. This may be partly due to the tendency by medical certifiers to record pneumonia as the underlying cause of death of the elderly. But it also may be because pneumonia has become more severe as drug-resistant microbes have arisen and new infections have appeared. It is caused by the bacteria *Streptococcus pneumoniae,* which can mutate and become resistant to some antibiotics.

In fact, pneumonia is now one of the most serious infections in elderly persons, especially among women and the oldest old. In a study of pneumonia patients who acquired the disease in nursing homes and were hospitalized, pneumonia resulted in the deaths of 40% of the patients (Centers for Disease Control and Prevention, 1997).

Septicemia is the sixth leading cause of death for black women 85 years of age and older but is less prevalent among other demographic groups. This disease is nonspecific and often begins with bacterial infections of the urinary tract, skin, or respiratory system.

Injuries are still a major cause of death among the elderly; though they kill a lower proportion of the elderly than they do of younger people, they lead to 2% of the deaths of those 65 years of age and older. Injuries from motor vehicle crashes, firearms, suffocation, and falls account for most deaths by injury.

Life Expectancy

Average life expectancy at birth increased from 47 years in 1900 to 77.8 years in 2005, but that is largely owing to better control of infant mortality. (A visit to any old cemetery shows a sad history of many deaths among infants, small children, and young women who died in childbirth.) The increase in life expectancy has had important effects on Medicare and other large programs that are dependent on age groups.

However, the typical human life span has not changed greatly. Even today, a person who reaches the age of 100 is considered extremely old. Cardiovascular disease, cancer, and other diseases still prevent most from reaching the century mark.

Is increasing the life span a worthwhile goal? Unless longer life is combined with good health, probably most people would prefer to die well before the age of 100. It is rare for anyone that old to retain the abilities to read, walk, converse, even to enjoy eating and drinking, which make life pleasurable. Despite those important considerations, some researchers continue to search for ways of prolonging the life span. Genetic engineering, surgery, and diet have all been involved in studies having the goal of postponing death. Currently, extreme calorie-restricted diets and the compound resveratrol (found in small amounts in grapes and red wine) are being used experimentally in animal and human subjects. They may lead to longer life, but the results with both methods are tentative.

A more fruitful approach for researchers on aging may be to search for ways to counteract the effects of aging so that our last years—whatever their length—can be satisfying ones. Already many elderly are being helped to feel or look better with cosmetic surgery, drugs for arthritis and osteoporosis, nutrition, and exercise. Some of these remedies also can provide protection from cardiovascular disease and cancer, the diseases that are most likely to shorten lives or cause years of suffering.

Physical and emotional health in the elderly benefit from social contacts. Having a network of friends and acquaintances is important for many reasons, including the ability to call on other people for occasional help. Marriage, especially, has a great impact on health: In a large study of the elderly and how their marital status affects health, Schone and Weinick (1998) found that both men and women have healthier behaviors (related to eating, drinking alcohol, and exercising) if they are married than if they are single. The beneficial effect was more pronounced for men than women.

At all ages, having a good sense of humor enriches life and may prolong it. As journalist Norman Cousins made famous in his *Anatomy of an Illness* (1979), watching old Marx Brothers movies aided him greatly in recovering from cardiovascular disease. He later became a lecturer at medical schools, helping doctors understand the importance of humor.

CHAPTER 2

Overview of Geriatric Health Information

This chapter provides general information about health in the elderly. Information about specific diseases can be found in Part II.

CIRCULATION

As blood moves through the arteries and veins, it creates pressure against the blood vessels' walls. Each time the heart contracts, it causes the blood pressure to be the greatest. This pressure is called the systolic pressure. When the heart relaxes, the pressure falls to the lowest level, called the diastolic pressure. The numbers are shown as a systolic/diastolic ratio; for example, a systolic blood pressure of 115 and a diastolic blood pressure of 75 is shown as 115/75. Normal systolic blood pressure is usually characterized as being less than 120, and normal diastolic blood pressure, as less than 80.

Elderly people may be given these guidelines for determining what their blood pressure signifies:

- If one's systolic pressure is usually 120 to 139, and the diastolic pressure is usually 80 to 89, that is prehypertension. The person may feel well, as there are no symptoms. However, hypertension may develop if the person smokes or fails to use diet and exercise.
- In Stage 1 hypertension, the systolic pressure is usually 140 to 159, and the diastolic pressure is usually 90 to 99. In addition to making important lifestyle changes, the person may need to take at least one medicine.

• Systolic pressure is usually 160 or more, and diastolic pressure is usually 100 or more in Stage 2 hypertension. In addition to making important lifestyle changes, a person in this stage may need to take two or more medicines.

NUTRITION AND EXERCISE

If good nutrition and exercise are important for the young, they are vital for the elderly. Elderly retired people may be more able to manage these aspects of health than when they were younger. After retirement from full-time employment, they have more time for exercise and meal planning. Also, after some of their acquaintances die or become ill from preventable illnesses, they realize the importance of giving up smoking, limiting alcohol, eating intelligently, and exercising.

Many people eat less as they age, which is likely to lead to malnourishment unless they are extremely careful to get the proper balance of nutrients, vitamins, and minerals. Similarly, as a person's joints stiffen, he is apt to walk and exercise less. However, continued movement is essential for maintaining strength, balance, flexibility, and endurance. In addition, good nutrition and exercise help people to sleep soundly and to avoid mild depression.

Body mass index (BMI) gives a good indication of whether a person is at a desirable weight. Obesity is defined as a BMI of at least 30. If a popula-

---

BMI

BMI is calculated as follows:

Weigh yourself. Your weight = _____ pounds.

Your weight in pounds ÷ 2.2 = _____ weight in kilograms.

Measure your height in inches. Your height = _____ inches.

Your height in inches ÷ 39.4 = _____ height in meters.

Your weight in kilograms / (height in meters)^2 = _____ = BMI.

For example, a person who is 5 feet 7 inches and weighs 140 pounds has a BMI of 22. An easier way of finding your BMI is to use a BMI table; many are available online. Or, use the AARP's Web site, http://www.aarp.org/health/fitness/info-05-2010/bmi_calculator.html, to enter your height and weight and have your BMI calculated automatically.

tion's mortality rate is graphed along with BMI, the very lowest and highest BMIs are associated with the highest mortality rates.

Fat distribution is also important. Accumulation of fat around the waist, resulting in an "apple" shape, raises the risk of stroke, diabetes, hypertension, and coronary artery disease more than accumulation of fat in the lower body (the "pear" shape) does.

Losing weight can be difficult at any age. Groups such as Weight Watchers and Overeaters Anonymous are often helpful, providing some socialization as well as advice and support for those who need to lose weight.

Dehydration is a frequent problem for the elderly, partly because they simply forget to drink water unless they feel thirsty. Drinking about eight cups of water or watery liquids a day helps a variety of conditions, such as hypertension, mental confusion, and constipation. Remembering to drink is easier if the person makes a habit of drinking water with each meal and with medicines. Water is often more palatable if a carafe is kept in the refrigerator, so that it is chilled and gases in it can evaporate.

In the past, vitamin D deficiency was the cause of rickets in children and of osteomalacia in adults who had too little access to animal protein and fortified milk. Even now, it is linked by some researchers to a variety of disorders—osteoporosis, weakened muscles, bone fractures, various types of cancer, autoimmune diseases, diabetes, schizophrenia, depression, and cardiovascular diseases—and is rather easy to remedy. About 15 to 20 minutes per day of exposure to moderate sunlight enables the body to manufacture a therapeutic dose of vitamin D. When that is not possible, vitamin D supplements can be taken. Natural sources of vitamin D are fatty fish such as herring and salmon, cod liver oil, beef liver, and eggs. Many foods are now fortified with vitamin D. Flour, milk, breakfast cereals, bread, yogurt, and margarine often contain vitamin D. Sunlight is often blamed for skin cancer, and overexposure to sunlight is dangerous; but sometimes people spend too little time in sunlight and become deficient in vitamin D.

A Mediterranean-type diet appears to be good for general health and to help those who need to lose weight. It emphasizes eating fish, olive oil, legumes, fresh vegetables and fruits, and little meat or dairy foods. Small amounts of wine are an optional addition.

Eating can be difficult if a person's teeth are in bad condition, and in the past many of the elderly lost their teeth. In recent years, better dental care has been available, people floss their teeth more, and they are more likely to have their teeth X-rayed and checked by a dental hygienist or dentist than people were at one time. As a result, more of the elderly are keeping their natural teeth.

Because they anchor the teeth, the gums are extremely important. If plaque builds up beneath the gum line, it can cause infection. Gum disease, called gingivitis, makes the gums tender, and they may bleed. If gingivitis or other gum diseases are serious, they may have to be treated by a dentist or dental surgeon. In the early stages of gum disease, the gums can be repaired by daily brushing and flossing. Later, gum disease can lead to infections that ruin the teeth, the gums, and even the bones underlying the gums, so that the teeth must be removed.

Good dentures and dental implants can help greatly if the natural teeth cannot be saved. However, implants are very expensive and may not be covered by health insurance. Both for effectiveness and for containing cost, it is highly desirable for elderly people to keep their natural teeth rather than to replace them with dentures or implants.

Daily care that helps elderly people keep their teeth and gums healthy includes twice-daily flossing and brushing (of the tongue as well as the teeth) with fluoride toothpaste, regular checkups and cleaning by a dentist, good nutrition, and avoidance of smoking.

Dryness of the mouth was once thought to be a natural consequence of aging, but now it is known that dry mouth is usually the result of disease or medication. Normal salivation can help lubricate chewed food, making it easier to swallow the food and to begin digesting it. Dry mouth can lead to tooth decay, also. Those who do have dry mouth can help the condition by sipping water or sugarless drinks, avoiding caffeine and alcohol, and not smoking.

Like the rest of the skin, the lips and tongue may become drier and thinner in an elderly person. Tobacco use, broken teeth, or badly fitting dentures can lead to a thickening of the skin lining the mouth, and the tongue may develop fissures and enlarged veins. Some teeth may be chipped if a person grinds her teeth or has poor nutrition.

If the teeth are badly damaged, partial or full dentures may be necessary. Dentures are made to fit the person's mouth and (if partial) to match the remaining teeth. Even so, they may not fit well at first and will need to be adjusted or replaced. At best, they are uncomfortable, even with improved chewing ability, reinforcing the importance of caring for one's natural teeth. Eating with dentures is difficult at first; the patient should start with small pieces of soft food, chew slowly, and be careful. Wearing the dentures may interfere with the wearer's ability to feel hot foods and liquids or to sense bones or other sharp objects in food. Daily cleaning of dentures keeps them clean and free of stains and protects against swollen gums and bad breath. Dentures should be brushed daily with a special denture-care product and placed in water or a denture-cleansing liquid at night.

Exercise is as important as nutrition for maintaining health in the elderly. However, it should be appropriate for a person's age and physical condition and should be approved by a doctor. Even taking a treadmill test can be stressful for someone who has some atherosclerosis or other circulatory problems.

Walking for at least half an hour daily is often necessary for the elderly, providing good aerobic exercise (exercise that increases the rate of metabolism by increasing oxygen consumption) and costing nothing. Even that amount of exercise is useful for weight control and for avoiding mild depression. Some elderly people like walking in shopping malls or other places where they feel safe and can walk on a smooth surface; others prefer walking on a trail through a forest or around a lake. Walking can be adapted to many preferences and environments and can be a solitary or companionable activity. Some warm-up stretches are often recommended before walking, though some recent research shows they are not needed.

Swimming is another excellent exercise, especially for those who have joint pain and cannot walk or perform other weight-bearing exercises. Though swimming laps provides maximum benefit, some people cannot swim well enough to do laps; they can do aquatic exercises, however, if they have access to a swimming pool.

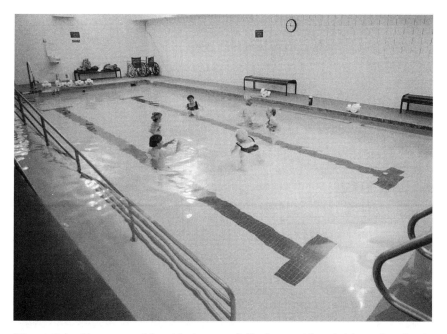

Figure 2.1   For many of the elderly, especially those with arthritis, swimming is an excellent exercise. (AP Photo/Murrae Haynes.)

A stationary bike or treadmill can also provide aerobic exercise. The monotony of using such machines can be relieved with music or reading, and they are invaluable when the weather makes it impossible to exercise outdoors. Anyone can begin with a few minutes of cycling or walking at a slow speed and gradually increase the time and pace.

Upper-body strength is increased by lifting free weights. Over time, the number of repetitions and heaviness of the weights can be increased. Weight lifting increases muscle mass without increasing oxygen consumption and is thus an anaerobic exercise.

A study of 100 frail residents of a nursing home who were aged 72 to 98 showed the benefits of resistance strength training, using a leg press (Flatarone et al., 1994). The residents were divided into four groups for the study, which lasted 10 weeks:

- Group 1 used a leg press for regular resistance strength training.
- Group 2 was given multinutrient supplements.
- Group 3 used a leg press for regular resistance strength training and was given multinutrient supplements.
- Group 4 (the control group) received neither multinutrient supplements nor strength training.

Those who exercised increased their muscle strength 113%. In addition, the pace of their walking increased 12%. In the nonexercisers, walking pace declined 1%. The exercisers' stair-climbing power increased by 28%, and their overall level of physical activity increased. The multinutrient supplements had no effect on any of the outcomes.

Another anaerobic exercise is provided by tai chi chih, a variation of tai chi that is especially beneficial for the elderly. Most of the movement depends on the leg muscles, which are strengthened by the activity. Tai chi chih also helps some people with equilibrium, hypertension, and even urinary incontinence. Many of its practitioners meditate while doing tai chi chih, which also leads to relaxation and calmness. Although books and compact discs showing tai chi chih can be used, it is best learned from a well-qualified instructor. The official Web site is http://www.taichi chih.org.

Some seniors are able to go beyond these basic exercises—to take strenuous hikes, for example. If they take reasonable precautions for safety and physical stress, the activity can greatly help them stay healthy and avoid depression.

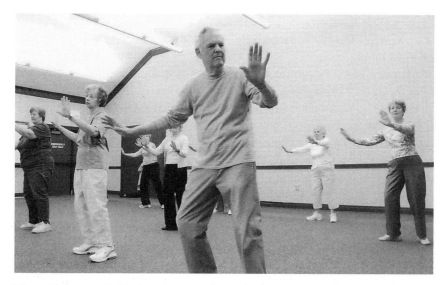

Figure 2.2 A tai chi class for older adults. (AP Photo/University of Southern Mississippi, Steve Rouse.)

THE MUSCLES AND SKELETON

Most aging people are well aware of the dangers of cancer and cardio-vascular diseases, but most of the pain and disability in those over age 65 is related to the decline of the skeleton and muscles (Dieppe and Tobias, 1998). As we age, our movements become less fluid and more painful. In the most serious cases, osteoporosis can cause fractures.

Most people, as they age, find that physical activity becomes more difficult. Even the most athletic people can no longer play tennis, run marathons, or play ball as they did when they were younger. Those who were less active in their youth may find even walking painful: Back and neck pain are common, and movements become stiff. Osteoarthritis is very common; it afflicts two-thirds of the over-55 population. People who had rheumatoid arthritis or musculoskeletal trauma when they were young have even more pain and disability as they age. All these changes are related to changes in the skeleton and muscles. The connective tissues change as we age, also. Calcium crystals may form, leading to painful joint disorders.

Age-related changes in the skeleton are the result of changes at the cellular level. Osteoclasts are cells that cause resorption of bone. Their activity increases with a person's age. Meanwhile, the activity of osteoblasts (which make bone) lessens, especially in postmenopausal women. (Estrogen inhibits the effect of osteoclasts, and, to a lesser degree, androgens do also.) If more bone is resorbed than formed, the skeleton becomes weaker and more likely to break.

Estrogen has a large effect on bone density, which begins to decrease after the age of 30. Because the level of estrogen naturally falls in women around the age of menopause, bone density also dwindles. Ultimately, a woman may develop osteoporosis. In this condition, the total amount of bone decreases, and the skeleton is thin and filled with spaces. Although osteoporosis in postmenopausal women is well known, it also can occur in men. Whites and Asians are more likely than others to develop it, and the risk rises greatly after about the age of 50. Women who do not take estrogen after menopause are also more vulnerable, as are men and women who use steroids for more than three months.

Bone is made largely of collagen, which provides tensile strength, and hydroxyapatite, which gives bone its rigidity. Hydroxyapatite is a large molecule that contains much calcium and phosphorus. Thus, some of the effects of aging on the skeleton can be opposed by a good diet. Even in the young, drinking milk helps form and preserve bone by providing calcium and phosphate. For those who are lactose-intolerant or vegetarian, those minerals can be provided in supplements. Exercise is also important: Weight-bearing exercises such as running or rapid walking are helpful. Weight control is helpful; bones and joints can support a lightweight person much more easily than a heavy one. Because older persons have a higher proportion of fat and a lower proportion of muscle than when they were younger, most people need to lose weight as they age.

The group of vitamins known collectively as vitamin D affects bone composition. The two major members of the group are ergocalciferol (vitamin D_2) and cholecalciferol (vitamin D_3). When neither type is specified, the term vitamin D can mean either or both of these substances. Sunlight activates a precursor in the skin, changing it to vitamin D. As it travels throughout the body, the vitamin is gradually modified to the hormone calcitriol. Calcitriol defends the body against some bacteria and helps to regulate the concentrations of phosphate and calcium—the elements needed for making bone—in the circulatory system.

In the past, vitamin D deficiency was the cause of rickets in children and of osteomalacia in adults who had too little access to animal protein and fortified milk. Even now, it is linked by some researchers to a variety of disorders—osteoporosis, weakened muscles, bone fractures, various types of cancer, autoimmune diseases, diabetes, schizophrenia, depression, and cardiovascular diseases—and is rather easy to remedy. About 15 to 20 minutes per day of exposure to moderate sunlight enables the body to manufacture a therapeutic dose of vitamin D. When that is not possible, vitamin D supplements can be taken. Natural sources of vitamin D are fatty fish such as herring and salmon, cod liver oil, beef liver, and eggs. Many foods are now fortified with vitamin D. Flour, milk, breakfast cereals, bread, yogurt, and margarine often contain vitamin D. Sunlight is often blamed for skin cancer, and overexposure to sunlight is dangerous; but sometimes people spend too little time in sunlight and become deficient in vitamin D.

FOOT CARE

Foot care is especially important for diabetic persons and for anyone with circulatory problems. The feet must be kept clean and dry to prevent skin damage. Moisturizing creams combat dry skin that may become fragile, crack, and bleed. Damage to the feet is not only painful but also can allow bacteria to enter the skin and cause infections.

Many conditions that are common in elderly people can lead to foot problems, which afflict about 70% of those over age 65. In addition to diabetes, the conditions include arthritis of various kinds, cardiovascular disease, and osteoporosis.

Even for those with good circulation, the feet can be a source of discomfort or pain. The elderly with foot problems are also likely to avoid walking, and so they lose the healthful effects of exercise.

Feet may be deformed in elderly people who have arthritis or have worn ill-fitting shoes. Elderly women who wore shoes with spike heels and pointed toes when they were young may now have bunions and toes that are curved and crowded tightly together. Only surgery can help in many cases, though wearing larger shoes, cushioning toes, and separating the toes with lamb's wool can greatly increase a person's comfort. Other conservative measures that can alleviate painful foot conditions include rest, nonsteroidal anti-inflammatory drugs (NSAIDs), and corticosteroid injections.

The podiatrist is thus an important member of the geriatrics team. He can examine the feet externally for bunions, calluses, and corns and can examine the muscles and bones of the feet with X-rays. Podiatrists have the degree of doctor of podiatric medicine. They can perform minor surgery and prescribe drugs or physical therapy that can help patients.

SMOKING

Chemicals in tobacco pass through the lungs and into the bloodstream of smokers and soon reach the heart, which then beats more forcefully and speedily. At the same time, the blood vessels constrict, and the passages are narrowed. These changes lead to hypertension (high blood pressure). In addition, the narrowed blood vessels are more likely to be blocked by a clot. Smoking also lowers the amount of high-density ("good") lipoprotein in the blood and leads to atherosclerosis, or the buildup of plaques in the vessels. Taken all together, these alterations in the blood raise the smoker's risk of a myocardial infarction (heart attack) or stroke.

Some elderly people assume that if they have been smoking most of their lives, the physical damage is done, they have an addiction that is hard to break, and they may as well continue the habit. However, research has shown that it is never too late to quit smoking. Significant results can be seen within a year. Anyone who stops smoking is likely to live longer; to have a lower risk of cancer, heart attack, osteoporosis, emphysema, or lung cancer; and to have better blood circulation.

Aside from those effects, smokers set a poor example for their children and grandchildren, who are more likely to begin smoking themselves and may be harmed by breathing secondhand smoke. In a study of 405 children who underwent outpatient surgery, it was found that, in addition to the direct effects of exposure to secondhand smoke, the children who lived with smokers had many more complications of surgery than those who did not live with smokers (Jones and Bhattacharyya, 2006). Some of the children had to use bronchodilators following surgery; others had to be hospitalized overnight. In the recovery room, some choked, gagged, or secreted fluids into the respiratory tract.

Most longtime smokers are addicted to the nicotine in tobacco products, and breaking the addiction can be extremely difficult. Withdrawal symptoms such as headaches may occur, especially during the first few weeks after quitting. The most important step one can take is to decide to stop smoking on a certain date; after that, a variety of helps may be needed. These differ with the individual. Some people simply stop cold turkey; others may join support groups or use nicotine replacements or medicines that help ease the withdrawal symptoms.

Pipe and cigar smokers and users of chewing tobacco or snuff should be aware that, like cigarette smokers, they are in danger from tobacco. They may develop cancer of the mouth, bladder, lungs, and other parts of the body. In addition, they are endangering those around them with secondhand smoke, which can cause or worsen respiratory diseases.

DRUGS

Elderly patients tend to take more drugs than younger people and to react to them differently. Not surprisingly, they also have more adverse drug reactions. Though effective drugs for many conditions have proliferated and are welcomed by physicians and their patients, it is well to be aware of potential pitfalls in drug use (Woodson, 1998).

In some cases, drugs may not be needed at all. Some conditions can be prevented or controlled by changes in lifestyle or other nondrug treatments:

- High cholesterol level may be lowered by a low-fat diet
- Type 2 diabetes may be controlled by diet and exercise
- Depression may respond to psychotherapy
- Elevated blood pressure may be lowered by reducing alcohol and salt, losing weight, and exercising
- Imbalance in walking can be helped by exercise or by using a cane or walker
- Insomnia may lessen with dietary or behavioral changes
- Arthritis may respond to physical therapy or transcutaneous electrical nerve stimulation

Not only can some of these treatments help the specific conditions and avoid overuse of drugs, but they may have a general beneficial effect on the patient's body. Most physicians tend to recommend trying these measures before taking drugs.

When drugs must be used, they should be chosen carefully and the dosage made appropriate to the patient. Often elderly persons need a smaller amount of a medicine than younger persons, because their kidneys or livers remove less of the drug from the blood. For example, as they age, many people find that they become less tolerant of alcohol. They may drink the same amount as when they were younger, but it leads to a higher concentration of alcohol in their bloodstream. They become drunk or have a hangover the next day after drinking only a small amount.

Body composition also affects what happens to drugs. With age, the proportion of body fat increases and that of body water decreases. The change in body fat tends to prolong the effect of some drugs, so an older patient may not have to take a drug as often as a younger patient has to. The lower proportion of water in the body leads to a higher concentration of drugs; thus, a lower dosage may be needed for the elderly.

Drug level also may increase in the elderly as a result of blood protein levels. Many older people have a lower level of serum albumin, which can raise the level of a drug.

Another difficulty with medicating the elderly is the potential for drug interactions. Many patients have several conditions for which they may be taking drugs, and physicians need to use caution in prescribing additional ones.

Some drugs—especially sedatives—can magnify the problems elderly patients already tend to have, such as falling. Some diuretics and other drugs for hypertension can lead to dizziness or lightheadedness.

A small percentage of any group using any drugs will have adverse reactions. For example, diuretics—often prescribed for hypertension—can lead to dehydration or hypotension (low blood pressure). Other drugs can cause rashes or damage the liver or kidneys. The printed information that accompanies a prescription has valuable information about possible adverse reactions and should be read carefully when a patient takes a drug for the first time. It is obviously important for patients to be aware of possible adverse reactions and to report any that occur to their physicians immediately.

For all these reasons, drugs must be administered with caution in older patients. Usually, but not always, the initial dosage should be small. But merely reducing the dosage of drugs in the elderly is not sufficient. Continual monitoring by the patient and physician is important. If a drug is ineffective at an initial low dosage, it may be necessary to increase the dosage or to try another medicine. Also, a patient may become frail or develop a new illness requiring a different drug.

Given all of this, it might seem that drugs cause more problems than they solve. However, despite all the potential problems associated with drugs, they can be lifesaving for the elderly as well as for the general population.

The following table shows various drugs that are commonly prescribed for disorders affecting many elderly patients. Though many are better known by trade names (such as Plavix, a trade name for clopidogrel), for consistency and comparison, the names shown here are generic. When first introduced, a drug is protected legally from competition; after the patent expires (generally in 20 years, but the period is variable), other pharmaceutical companies can produce the same generic drug under their own trade names. So, a generic medicine may be available from several companies under different trade names. It can also be sold under the generic name, and it is usually less costly when it is sold that way.

Pharmaceutical companies spend a great deal of money on advertising to create the impression that their trademarked drugs are superior to the generic versions. However, in general, a drug sold under its generic name is no less effective, and no more likely to cause adverse reactions, than the same drug sold under one of its trade names.

Many elderly people take a variety of prescription and over-the-counter medications to prevent or treat atherosclerosis and other conditions. Some drug combinations can occasionally lead to problems, such as decreased

Table 2.1 Drugs That Are Often Prescribed for the Elderly

Generic Drug	Medical Use	Action
Amiodarone	Rapid heart beat	Affects the heart's electrical system that governs cardiac muscle contraction
Verapamil, amlodipine, diltiazem CD	High blood pressure, angina, cardiac arrhythmias	Calcium channel blocker (slows the movement of calcium ions into muscle cells)
Lisinopril	High blood pressure, congestive heart failure	ACE (angiotensin converting enzyme) inhibitor (relaxes arteries and increases excretion of water by kidneys)
Terazosin	High blood pressure and benign prostatic hyperplasia (enlarged prostate)	Alpha-adrenergic blocker (causes blood vessels to relax and expand, improving blood flow). Relaxes muscles in the prostate and bladder neck, making urination easier
Digoxin	Congestive heart failure, atrial fibrillation	Helps the heart beat more strongly and with a more regular rhythm
Hydrochlorothiazide	High blood pressure, edema	Diuretic (prevents body from absorbing salt; increases urination)
Warfarin	Prevention of blood clotting	Inhibits clumping of platelets in blood
Oxybutynin	Urinary incontinence	Antispasmodic
Donepezil	Alzheimer's disease	Improves the functioning of nerve cells in the brain by preventing the breakdown of acetylcholine

(Continued)

Table 2.1 (*Continued*)

Generic Drug	Medical Use	Action
Clopidogrel	Atherosclerotic cardio-vascular disease	Inhibits clumping of platelets in blood that can lead to blood clots
Statins (various names ending in -*statin*)	High cholesterol level	Improve blood cholesterol levels, especially reducing low-density lipoprotein levels
Atenolol, propranolol	High blood pressure, glaucoma, migraines	Beta blockers, or beta-adrenergic blocking agents, block the effects of the hormone epinephrine (adrenaline). The heart beats more slowly and less forcefully, reducing blood pressure. Beta blockers also help blood vessels expand to improve blood flow.
Meloxicam	Osteoarthritis, fever, inflammation	An NSAID that blocks the enzymes that make prostaglandins and lowers the level of prostaglandins

effectiveness (from the combination of albuterol and atenolol); hyperkalemia, or too much potassium in the blood, which can lead to heart arrhythmia (from the combination of lisinopril and potassium); risk of bleeding (from the combination of aspirin and warfarin); and risk of muscle damage (from the combination of niacin and some statins). Although physicians and pharmacists should be aware of these risks and advise patients to avoid risky combinations, the patients may not think of mentioning the over-the-counter medicines, herbal remedies, alcohol, and dietary supplements they are using along with their prescriptions. For safety, it is important for patients to make their physicians aware of all substances they are using. In a 2006 study of 3,305 men and women aged 57 to 85, researchers found that 4% were at risk of a major drug interaction; half of them involved nonprescription medications (Qato et al., 2008).

It is fairly common for elderly people to have many illnesses and to receive a different medication for each one. For instance, they may suffer from diabetes, chronic obstructive pulmonary disease, hypertension, osteoporosis, and osteoarthritis. Some postmenopausal women take estrogen to relieve the symptoms of menopause, and many men and women take statin drugs for the prevention of heart disease. People may take 15 or 20 pills and capsules a day, even if they are relatively healthy. Monitoring all these drugs and their possible interactions is extremely difficult for a physician who may be limited to spending 15 minutes on each patient visit. As a safeguard, patients should take responsibility for keeping track of all medications. Pharmacists, as well as physicians, can answer many questions about possible side effects and the risks of combining various drugs.

ALCOHOL

Drinking alcohol in moderation is widespread and accepted in U.S. culture. A glass of wine or beer with friends or family can be one of life's little pleasures, and recent research even tells us that a little red wine is beneficial to the cardiovascular system. Considering the risk of heart disease for older people, it may seem that they should continue drinking wine, or even begin doing so if they have not used alcohol previously. However, the elderly need to be especially cautious about limiting their drinking. Although some elderly people can drink without adverse consequences, and may even benefit from a daily glass of red wine, others need to lower their alcohol consumption. They should not drink at the same level as when they were young, because their tolerance has decreased. (Blood alcohol concentration is increased by 20% in elderly people.) They also should not take powerful drugs that cannot be used safely with alcohol. Many elderly take a variety of medicines for cardiovascular conditions, arthritis, and other disorders that were not available until recent years.

Depression, lack of social contacts, and loneliness are the usual precursors to alcohol abuse in the elderly. After they retire or become widowed, they are in special danger. Becoming involved in taking classes, doing paid or volunteer work, or taking part in other activities can help protect the elderly from turning to alcohol for comfort.

At what point does moderate drinking become alcohol abuse? Like other medical questions for the elderly, the answer depends on the individual. The National Institute on Alcohol Abuse and Alcoholism defines hazardous use of alcohol for those aged 65 and older as three or more drinks at a sitting, or more than seven drinks in a week (Blow, 1998). Moderate use is defined as one drink—4 or 5 ounces of wine, 12 ounces of beer, or a shot

(1.5 ounces) of liquor—daily. Some of the elderly are able to scale back the amount or type of alcohol they consume and avoid problems. However, a study by the Centers for Disease Control and Prevention (2007) found that 5.9% of all men over the age of 60 and 0.9% of all women in that age group reported monthly or more frequent binge drinking.

While younger alcohol abusers usually consume alcohol in social settings, most elderly abusers drink while alone at home, which can lead to accidents and lack of interest in more rewarding activities. Falls are common in the elderly anyway, and use of alcohol can increase falls. The falls themselves are more serious in the elderly, who may have osteoporosis and other conditions that increase the damaging effects of falls.

Age-related decline in mental function can increase because of alcohol use. Chronic alcohol consumption can damage parts of the brain that are essential for thinking. In addition to the direct effect on cognition, this can interfere with self-monitoring of alcohol use.

The Centers for Disease Control study (2007) covered the period 1997 through 2001. With the aging of the baby boomers, who reached adulthood during the years of more relaxed attitudes toward drugs, there may be an increase in abuse of alcohol and other drugs. Because the oldest baby boomers reached the age of 60 in 2006, any increase should soon become apparent.

Some of those who become alcoholics after becoming elderly—who as a group are more affluent, more likely to be women, and more likely to have increased their drinking after a stressful major event—face relatively few medical problems. In other cases, an elderly person may have been an alcoholic for many years. These people tend to have more severe problems than those who become dependent on alcohol late in life.

No one wants to face the possibility of being an alcoholic. The slide from moderate social drinking to alcoholism can be very gradual, and the effects may be unnoticed. A retiree does not lose time from work or fail to meet obligations that would be red flags in a younger person. Physicians may fail to question patients about alcohol use, assuming that a person who appears in control of their life has no issues with drinking. In fact, alcohol use is so common in U.S. culture that asking patients whether they drink does not occur to many doctors. Formal screening for alcohol problems is used by only 13% of primary care physicians (Di Bari et al., 2002). Often a family member or friend must be the one to notice a serious problem and to prod the person to seek help.

Free or low-cost support groups can help any alcoholic recover. The best known group is Alcoholics Anonymous (AA; www.aa.org). AA tends to emphasize a spiritual approach, with the members encouraged to lean on some higher power for help. The founders pioneered a 12-step approach to addiction now used by a variety of support groups. The steps include admitting lack of control over an addiction, recognizing a greater power that can give strength, examining and making amends for past errors, and providing help for other addicts. AA was originally founded by Christians who stressed reliance on Jesus, but over the years it has become less obviously Christian.

Another group is the more secular LifeRing (www.unhooked.com), which is more appealing to many who prefer a humanistic and supportive, but less religious, approach to their problem. It was founded to give people an alternative to AA. The LifeRing Web site proclaims, "LifeRing supports recovery methods that rely on human efforts rather than on divine intervention or faith-healing."

In addition, many hospitals, churches, and temples have support groups that may be open to the general public. A common thread among all these groups is that members assist each other, which may help the social isolation that can promote drinking in the elderly.

Online help is available, also. For instance, AA's Web site shows a useful list of 12 questions for prospective members to ask themselves to determine whether they need help with alcoholism. LifeRing's Web site includes online meetings for members.

Both AA and LifeRing accept and offer support to people suffering from other drug addictions, such as addiction to pain medications or sleep aids. AA has several specialized groups, and LifeRing meetings may have members with different kinds of addiction.

Because none of the groups exert pressure on prospective members to continue attending, anyone who suspects they may be drinking too much can attend a meeting or two for more information and for feedback about their drinking habits. Some can be reassured that their drinking is moderate and age-appropriate; others may need to give up alcohol altogether and can find the support they need.

A respectful attitude, coupled with a supportive environment, can help elderly alcoholics recover. Confrontational approaches have been used traditionally, but they may be inappropriate for many elderly people. In a program of the U.S. Department of Veterans Affairs for older alcoholics, researchers found that developing patient self-esteem and peer relationships were especially useful (Kashner et al., 1992).

SEXUALITY

Like other physical and mental activities, the sexuality of aging people is affected by general health. However, sexual activity continues to an extent that may surprise the young. In a study of 2,005 U.S. adults between the ages of 57 and 85, it was found that 73% of those aged 57 to 64, 53% of those aged 65 to 74, and 26% of those 75 and over were sexually active. Those who were inactive might have benefited from counseling or medication, but of women over 50 having low desire for sex, only 22% reported discussing it with a doctor. Similarly, 38% of over-age-50 men having erectile dysfunction, or impotence, talked with a doctor about it (Lindau et al., 2007). Complicating the problem, some physicians are supportive of patients' wishes to remain sexually active but have little knowledge of how to advise the patients.

For both men and women who have partners, there may be physical barriers to intimacy. Erectile dysfunction, for example, makes it impossible for a man to maintain a penile erection that is firm enough for intercourse.

"Curing" erectile dysfunction is not necessary in most cases. If treatment fails to restore youthful functioning, the elderly should realize they can be happily sexual with simple attitudinal changes. Accepting a partial erection, couples can use fingers, tongues, and sex toys to bring about orgasms.

Women's reactions are most important for a man's recognition of his limitations. If a woman accepts that her lover has trouble in climaxing as he did when young, they can both enjoy what they *can* experience. All or nothing is a self-defeating stance.

Women, too, need to be realistic in their expectations about sex as they age. Using a lubricant (alone or with estrogen, if a physician prescribes it) can counteract the discomfort of vaginal dryness, and for some women, hormone replacement therapy may be appropriate. However, physical problems may be overshadowed by psychological barriers. When a woman looks in a full-length mirror and sees her drooping bustline and shrinking fanny, she may not want a man to see her naked, especially if he is not a partner who has aged along with her. She needs to keep a sense of humor about her changing body, act positively, and see things in proportion. A man who is attracted to an elderly woman does not expect her to have the slim, firm body of a young girl. If she is cheerful, energetic, and interested in him, he will respond to her. (Or, if he is critical of her aging body, she may be better off without him.)

A woman may want to enhance her physical attractiveness to bolster her self-confidence, which can make her more outgoing and appealing to men. Cosmetic surgery, flattering clothing, and makeup can all have their places in a woman's life. However, they will not restore youth. Exercising and dieting are more likely to make a woman healthy and attractive—sexually as well as in general.

Probably many more elderly people would be sexually active if they were given the opportunity. Sex is an important part of normal adult life, and the aging feel its loss. For women, especially, partners tend to disappear in later life. Men die at a younger average age than women, and most men prefer younger partners; this leaves elderly women with a shortage of potential men partners. Lesbians are more fortunate in this respect, because they are more likely to age together and continue their relationship. Heterosexual women who have no partners are left with abstinence or masturbation; for women who have very conservative views about sex, those alternatives can lead to feelings of frustration or guilt. Vibrators, explicit films and books, and other sexual aids are available both for those who have no partners and for couples who use them together. Once considered "dirty," they are now used by a broad spectrum of people, including the elderly.

For those who are sexually active, some caution is in order. Many of the elderly have never been concerned about sexually transmitted diseases (STDs) because they had lifelong partners. After years of monogamy, they may assume that they are in no danger. If they find new sexual partners late in life, however, they need to be aware of the possible risks: STDs are widespread in the general population; they are not restricted to lower-class or promiscuous people. Condoms are for use by older, as well as for younger, couples. However, a recent University of Chicago survey of single women aged 58 and older revealed that about 60% had not used a condom the last time they had sex with a partner (American Geriatrics Society Foundation on Aging, 2010). Elderly people who had only vaginal sex when they were young may now be experimenting with oral or anal sex, which also can lead to transmission of STDs, and they need to be aware of that danger.

Physicians also may need to be reminded that advising about sexual issues and screening for STDs may be needed by their elderly patients (American Geriatrics Society Foundation on Aging, 2010). STDs, especially herpes and the human papillomavirus, are increasingly found in older people; chlamydia, gonorrhea, HIV—the virus that causes AIDS—and syphilis are dangers as well. There may not be any obvious symptoms, and an elderly person may mistake a symptom of an STD for an effect of aging. Though discussing sexual backgrounds and testing can be awkward for people just beginning a relationship, that awkwardness pales in comparison to the danger of contracting AIDS or some other serious STD. The best protection against that result is for both partners to be tested before they become sexually involved.

Using condoms and lubricants can help guard against transmission of STDs. Lubricants can help prevent sores and scratches of the penis or vagina through which microbes can pass. Postmenopausal women are more vulnerable than younger women to contracting STDs, because their vaginal walls are thinner.

Estrogen. Lack of sexual desire, less elastic skin, and diminished vaginal secretions can interfere with an elderly woman's sex life, as can the body changes that make her feel unattractive. These all result from the decrease in estrogen that occurs at menopause. Until the past few years, postmenopausal women were commonly treated with hormone replacement therapy, but studies linking estrogen/progesterone combinations to cardiovascular disease and other disorders have frightened many physicians and patients away from using hormone replacement therapy. The use of estrogen alone seems to be safer (Stefanick, 2006), and many continue to use it for its sexual and other health benefits.

Testosterone. Men's testes produce the hormone testosterone, which brings about sperm production. In addition, testosterone helps maintain bone density, muscle mass and strength, fat distribution, red blood cell production, and sex drive.

The body's testosterone level is at its highest during adolescence and early adulthood. After about the age of 40, the level declines. The decrease is gradual in most men.

Naturally declining testosterone levels may not cause any symptoms, but men who have very low levels of testosterone because of disease or treatments do exhibit effects. Their bones can become lighter, and muscles become smaller and weaker. The proportion of fat in their body decreases. Along with decreased sexual function, there may be a loss of memory and changes in mood. Some men experience these effects even though they do not have unusually low levels of testosterone. Others, having low levels of testosterone, fail to have any symptoms.

In some cases, testosterone therapy can be beneficial. Testosterone replacement medications may be necessary for men who have very low levels of testosterone (hypogonadism). These medications are available as injections and in patches and gels.

Some men hope that taking testosterone may help them feel better as they age. Testosterone therapy can restore testosterone to a youthful level, but there may be no benefit to this. Healthy men who take testosterone can increase muscle mass, but in most studies they were no stronger. Also, there is no evidence that a higher testosterone level can lengthen the life span. The risks of testosterone therapy in men with normal testosterone levels are unknown.

Some women benefit from taking testosterone. Testosterone may be helpful in increasing libido in postmenopausal women, many of whom experience a loss of interest in sex. The drug Estratest, which combines testosterone and estrogen, has been used successfully by some women for that purpose, though it has never been approved for that use by the Food and Drug Administration (FDA). In fact, some groups have petitioned the FDA to ban any marketing of the drug.

COMING TO TERMS WITH AGING

Retirement brings the good life to some, the opposite to others. Freed of working for others, many begin working for themselves or immerse themselves in hobbies. There is time to relax, enjoy grandchildren, and travel. However, a happy retirement depends on having a modest amount of money—or, for some people, a great deal of money—and good health. Chronic diseases and failing hearing or vision can cause retirement to be an unhappy time.

Even for those who are healthy and financially secure, retirement marks the end of a major phase of life. Some may joke that "at least aging can't last forever," but that is scant comfort.

We come to terms with aging and death in a variety of ways, but they can be grouped as acceptance or denial. Some people "go gentle into that good night"; others "rage, rage against the dying of the light" (Thomas, 1952). Even the very early harbingers of death can cause panic for some. In our youth-oriented society, we may color the very first gray hairs, wear clothing made for young people long after we look good in it, have plastic surgery to erase wrinkles and sags. Though they may seem silly or amusing, some of these tactics can be useful (and justifiable) professionally and socially. If an elderly actress can continue playing middle-aged roles, or an elderly politician can better relate to younger voters, for instance, they may feel the results justify the trouble and expense.

However, some elderly people who voluntarily allow themselves to appear old feel a great sense of relief when they stop trying to look younger than they are. Accepting aging can bring a reduction in stress in other ways, too. The competition with others ceases. When we attend class reunions, we are more interested in how old classmates are getting along physically and emotionally than in who looks the most glamorous or who has the most money and possessions. If we have accumulated some wealth over the years, we may be happily sharing it with others rather than trying to increase it.

For some of the elderly, the golden years are greatly overrated. When a church in California had a Sunday service devoted to the topic of aging, several of the older members spoke persuasively about their greater wisdom with age, about their joy in watching their grandchildren learn, and about other satisfactions. Then one woman, suffering with a degenerative neural disease, declared that "getting old really sucks." She went on to say more about the sadness of being widowed, the difficulties and pain of dealing with her disease, and the feelings of hopelessness that can come of reflecting on the wars and poverty in the world. For her and many others, sugarcoating the tribulations of aging makes no sense.

For most people, aging is a bittersweet time, filled with some satisfactions and some regrets. Poet Ruth Levitan (2009) expressed her own feelings in this manner:

Indian Summer

I carry my climate with me now,
Muggy as a summer storm,
the unsettled weather
of changing seasons
dampens my skin,
reminds me I have survived
the prickly heat of childhood,
flush of first pubescence,
furnaces of passion.
This new heat
tells me that life
with all its hungers, angers, loves,
still glows, radiates,
burns within me.

PART II

Issues and Controversies

CHAPTER 3

Medical Issues

DISORDERS ASSOCIATED WITH AGING

Some diseases are found mainly in elderly people; others are found in all age groups but are more serious or must be treated differently in the elderly. In both cases, individualized treatment is important.

Despite all we can do to make our later years healthy and satisfying, nearly everyone becomes ill with chronic or acute conditions. The following sections discuss conditions that particularly afflict the elderly.

Atherosclerosis

The most important disease to afflict the elderly is atherosclerosis, the buildup of lipid deposits in the arteries that causes cardiovascular disorders. Atherosclerosis occurs in stages, beginning with damage to arterial linings from smoking, hypertension (high blood pressure), environmental toxins, and other causes. When low-density lipoproteins accumulate and platelets form a cap over them, plaques are formed. These plaques narrow the arteries and interfere with blood flow. If the coronary arteries are blocked, too little blood reaches the heart muscle, which can lead to a heart attack (myocardial infarction), chronic heart disease, cardiac failure, or arrhythmias; if too little blood reaches the brain, a stroke, transient ischemic attack, or dementia may result; if too little blood reaches the peripheral arteries, there may be intermittent claudication (limping caused by poor circulation to the legs), chronic ischemia (lack of blood supply), gangrene, or amputation; if the aorta is blocked, there may be an aneurysm.

Prevention seems to be the best defense against atherosclerosis. Vigorous exercise, a low-fat diet, control of diabetes or hypertension, and avoidance of smoking are all effective.

In recent years, cardiologists have tended to treat patients having narrowed arteries with a procedure called balloon angioplasty. The artery is widened by sending water into it with a catheter, much as a balloon is blown up. Then a stent (a tube made of wire mesh) is inserted to keep the artery from deflating again. The stent is coated with drugs. This invasive treatment has proved very effective for patients who are having a heart attack and those who have severe chest pain after exertion.

However, people who have narrowed arteries may not need this expensive and risky treatment. No research has shown that balloon angioplasty prevents heart attacks; it appears now that conservative treatments—diet, exercise, not smoking, and medicines that lower blood pressure and cholesterol levels—are just as effective (Hoenig et al., 2010). In addition, a stent can sometimes lead to the formation of a clot in a coronary artery.

There is similar news about bypass surgery, which has been a common treatment for coronary artery disease for many years. For most patients, a conservative treatment is as successful for preventing heart attacks as bypass surgery is. Surgery is still recommended for patients who have advanced disease of the left main coronary artery or severe angina.

Cancer

Uncontrolled cell growth can result in a tumor that may or not be malignant (cancerous). Cancer (or carcinoma) cells can continue multiplying, spread to organs outside those where they began, and cause great damage to the body. Of course, any abnormal growth or other cancer symptom should be evaluated quickly but without undue fear. A benign tumor is rarely life-threatening, does not spread to other parts of the body, and is likely to be easily removable by surgery.

When cancer is found, treatment should be approached judiciously. In many cases, it is useful to get a second opinion from another doctor. In fact, some insurance companies require a second opinion, or they will pay for a second opinion if the patient requests it.

Cancer can affect any part of the body, but the elderly are most likely to be burdened with breast and prostate cancer.

Breast Cancer   Although cardiovascular disease is the major killer of women, breast cancer is still a danger. Women born today in the United States have a 1 in 8 chance of being diagnosed with breast cancer during their lifetime. That risk increases with age (National Cancer Institute, 2007). Women who are 65 or older have a 63.8% chance of developing it during the remainder of their life.

Many benign conditions can cause discomfort or lumps in the breast. Fibrocystic breast disease and fibroadenomas, for instance, cause lumps.

These may cause great concern and unnecessary worry. In fibrocystic breast disease, there is blockage in the breast ducts, leading to a buildup of fluid. Fibroadenomas are rubbery lumps that arise from an overgrowth of connective and glandular tissue in the breast. If found during a breast self-examination or routine mammogram, they should be evaluated to eliminate the possibility of cancer.

If breast cancer is confined to the ducts, it is called noninvasive. If it breaks through the walls of the ducts and the lobules (milk-secreting structures) and moves into the surrounding breast tissue, it is called invasive. It is called metastatic only when it begins in the breast, then spreads to other organs.

Early detection and treatment of breast cancer greatly improves the chance of survival. In fact, on average, 89% of patients survive at least five years after their diagnosis. The chances of survival are less when cancer is discovered or treated late. Thus, monthly self-examination of the breasts and armpits is important for all women. (As important as mammograms are, women who perform self-examinations find a large proportion of breast cancers.) Any of the following symptoms should be called to a physician's attention immediately:

- A thickening or lump, or nipple tenderness or pain, that persists after a menstrual period
- A new lump
- A change in the breast skin or nipple, including redness or scaliness
- Bleeding or discharge from the nipple
- Thickening or swelling of the breast
- Dimpling, indentation, or puckering of the breast

Only a small proportion of breast cancers can be explained by age, genetics, ethnicity, or other risk factors. Certain groups, however, have higher rates of the disease. Among women aged 50, whites face the greatest risk, followed by African Americans and Asians. Hispanic women have the lowest risk. Breast cancer also is more likely in women who began menstruating when they were 12 or younger or who went through menopause at age 55 or older. Women who have had a hysterectomy that included removal of the ovaries have a lower risk.

Though white women have the highest rate of breast cancer, it is more likely to be diagnosed at an early stage, when it is more treatable, than it is for women of other ethnic groups. Regardless of ethnicity or socioeconomic status, early and appropriate treatment leads to higher rates of survival.

If a woman's breasts contain much connective or glandular tissue, her risk of breast cancer is greater than if her breasts have a higher proportion of fatty tissue. However, other factors may be responsible for the heightened risk.

The effect of breast-feeding on a woman's future cancer risk is not well understood. The studies have not been comparable, and their results have varied (Yang and Jacobsen, 2008).

Obesity is a risk factor for many types of cancer, including breast cancer. The effect is especially marked in postmenopausal women and in those who gained weight gradually over the years rather than having been overweight since girlhood. Before menopause, being overweight actually protects a woman from breast cancer (Cui, 2002).

No specific foods have been shown to influence breast cancer, but heavy consumption of alcohol and caffeine probably increase the risk. Studies suggest a connection between diet and breast cancer: The disease is less common in countries where the diet is low in fats, such as in the Mediterranean countries. The fats in fish, monounsaturated oils such as olive and canola, high-fiber foods, and legumes all have a somewhat protective effect. Conversely, diets containing red meat and other fats seem to increase cancer risk. When women immigrate to the United States from other countries, their risk increases and grows even larger if they remain 20 years or longer.

Exercise confers many benefits on health, and brisk walking, if done at least a few times every week, lowers the risk of breast cancer.

Environmental factors are commonly suspected of causing cancer, but studies designed to assess the effects of pollutants have failed to show that they lead to any increase in breast cancer. Silicone implants can interfere with reading standard mammograms, but they do not appear to raise the risk of breast cancer. As discussed on page 65, women who have taken estrogen–progesterone combinations do have a slightly increased risk of developing breast cancer. This is true for women who have used oral contraceptives as well as those who have used hormone combinations for relieving the symptoms of menopause.

Genetics is now known to play a role in some breast cancers. The genes BRCA1 and BRCA2 increase the risk of both breast cancer and ovarian cancer. However, most breast cancer occurs in women who do not have those genes, and having them does not inevitably lead to cancer. Also, other factors interact with the breast cancer genes to increase the risk. A woman can benefit from genetic testing that shows she carries either of the genes, because she can consider undergoing surgery or other preventive treatment. On the other hand, some women fear learning they have the genes, because the information can be used by insurance companies to deny coverage. Thus, the decision whether to be tested can be very difficult.

Ethnic groups differ in mortality rates from breast cancer: Since 1975, the mortality rate for white women has decreased, but it has increased for African American women. The reasons are unclear; access to care, poverty level, and education may be contributing factors.

There is good news about five-year survival rates. For nearly every age and ethnic group, the survival rates have increased. The five-year survival rate is 86% for women who are 65 or older. This survival rate is higher than that in younger women, which may be because breast cancer in elderly women tends to be less aggressive.

For decades, women have been urged to have mammograms every year or two. However, it may be that mammograms are not as useful as has been assumed. Some of the cancers that are found by mammography are so slow-growing that they will not affect health, even if left untreated. The Nordic Cochrane Center collaborative in Copenhagen analyzed data in 2006 and found that for every 2,000 women between the ages of 50 and 70 who are screened for 10 years, only one will be saved from death. Additionally, 10 of them will be overtreated. The report has led to a debate in Britain about recommendations to patients about screening. In the United States, some experts feel the benefits have been oversold, but others continue to recommend routine screening (Rabin, 2009).

Though the probability of getting breast cancer increases greatly after the age of 65, many experts feel routine screening of elderly women is inadvisable. That opinion is based partly on financial considerations arising from the Copenhagen and other studies. Given the high cost of mammograms, some think screening should be limited to those who are at a high risk of dying from breast cancer. If a woman has heart disease or other heart problems that are more likely to cause her death, then screening for breast cancer may be redundant. Also, some elderly women are too frail to withstand treatment for cancer, and many cancers in elderly patients are slow growing and unlikely to be fatal.

On the other hand, an individual elderly woman may well choose to continue routine annual mammograms if she is in a high-risk group for breast cancer but is generally healthy otherwise. She may think breast cancer is more likely than anything else to cause her death. Because Medicare covers most or all of the cost of routine screens, expense is probably not a major issue for her.

Once diagnosed, the first step in treating breast cancer is to assign it to a stage. The stages are summarized in Table 3.1 (National Cancer Institute, 2011).

If the cancer is invasive, usually a biopsy will be done to determine how far the cells have spread. Treatment options include surgery, chemotherapy, radiation, and hormonal treatment. Many patients receive a combination

Table 3.1 Stages of Breast Cancer

Stage	Size of Cancer	Area Affected	Five-Year Survival Rate
0	Small; confined to layer of cells where it began	Within ductal system	100%
I	2 centimeters diameter or smaller	Within breast tissue	98%
IIA	2 to 5 centimeters diameter	Within breast tissue	88%
IIB	2 to 5 centimeters diameter	Breast and axillary lymph nodes	76%
IIIA	Up to 5 centimeters diameter or more	Breast and lymph nodes under arm	56%
IIIB	Up to 5 centimeters diameter or more	Cancer has spread from breast to nearby tissues	49%
IV	Varies	Cancer has spread from breast to many tissues	20%

Source: National Cancer Institute, 2011.

of two or more types of treatment, depending on the cancer stage and the person's characteristics.

As with other decisions about treatment, the patient should be actively engaged and knowledgeable about the risks and benefits of various procedures. Though an oncologist can provide invaluable advice about what can and should be done to kill the cancer cells, no one but the patient can know how much she values her appearance, health, and lifestyle.

Surgery is aimed at removing cells from a local area. For solid tumors, this may be enough. For many years, a radical mastectomy was used in every case of breast cancer; the entire breast, some lymph nodes under the arm, and some chest muscle were removed. Today mastectomies are usually limited to the breast and, in some cases, the lymph nodes. In lumpectomies, even the breast is conserved, because surgery is limited to the tumor and some surrounding tissue. Studies of patients who received lumpectomies or mastectomies showed no significant difference in survival rates. Surgery may be followed by breast reconstruction if a woman feels it is important. Reconstruction can be done at the time of the original surgery or later, so the patient's decision can be postponed until a time that may be less emotionally difficult.

Like surgery, radiation therapy targets a specific area—in the case of breast cancer, the tumor. Radiation kills the cancer cells or shrinks the tumor's size. The reason radiation is so effective is that it damages rapidly dividing cells, such as cancer cells, much more than it damages other cells. Radiation is sometimes used alone for breast cancer. Often it is used with surgery or chemotherapy. Radiation reduces the recurrences of cancer and increases the survival rate. Although it is extremely effective against breast cancer, radiation therapy does have side effects. These include fatigue and skin redness or burns.

Chemotherapy, or treatment with drugs, is often used as a supplement to surgery or radiation. Unlike surgery or radiation, which target small areas, chemotherapy affects cells of the entire body. It acts on the DNA in cells to interfere with cell reproduction. The disadvantages of chemotherapy are well known: Patients may have vomiting and nausea, be fatigued, lose their hair, and experience very toxic side effects. High doses of the chemicals can damage bone marrow, which makes blood cells, and may have no benefit compared with low doses. Despite the side effects, chemotherapy continues to be used. Current research is designed to learn what genetic characteristics would make it possible to predict what drugs would be most useful for attacking the cancer cells so that chemotherapy could be limited.

The hormone estrogen can promote the growth of breast cancer cells in some women whose cancer is hormone-dependent. Drugs that lower the amount of estrogen in the blood or that block its effects can increase the survival rate for that group of women. Remarkably, some of these drugs— tamoxifen, for example—act like estrogen in other tissues. Thus, the beneficial effects of estrogen on bone and cholesterol level are maintained. Tamoxifen is especially effective when it is combined with radiation therapy. The side effects are much like those of menopause, but tamoxifen does not cause menopause to begin. In addition, some patients using tamoxifen develop endometrial cancer or blood clots.

Raloxifene (Evista) is a newer drug for acting against estrogen. It appears to be as effective as tamoxifen and to have fewer side effects (National Cancer Institute, 2011). Postmenopausal women may be able to use raloxifene to prevent estrogen-sensitive breast cancer. Raloxifene was originally an osteoporosis drug. Compared with tamoxifen, raloxifene was less effective in preventing invasive breast cancer but more effective against noninvasive breast cancer. Both drugs work by interfering with the ability of estrogen to fuel tumor growth. Raloxifene caused fewer side effects and had a lower likelihood of causing uterine cancer than did tamoxifen. In addition, many women are already taking raloxifene to help maintain bone density and reduce the risk of vertebral fractures. That gives them a two-for-one reason to use raloxifene. On the other hand, tamoxifen stays in the body longer, which offers protection for a longer time after women stop taking the drug. A drug that lowers estrogen production, letrozole (Femara) has proved very effective in preventing recurrence of breast cancer in postmenopausal women who had been treated with tamoxifen.

The factors that can affect risk of developing invasive breast cancer are included in the Breast Cancer Risk Assessment Tool, an interactive program that can be found online at http://www.cancer.gov/bcrisktool/. After entering data about her family history, ethnicity, previous surgeries, and other factors, a woman receives an assessment of her personal risk.

Prostate Cancer   The benefit of routine screening is in doubt for prostate cancer as well as for breast cancer. Although prostate cancer is serious and often leads to death within the life span of a middle-aged man, in some cases, elderly patients may be able to avoid the surgery or radiation that is used to treat it. Whether such procedures are necessary depends on the patient's age, the prostate-specific antigen (PSA) level when the cancer is found, and the results of microscopic examination of the tumor.

Prostate cancer is very common in elderly men, and early detection and treatment is important. (In 2010, there were 217,730 new cases and 32,050 deaths in the United States.) The stages are summarized in Table 3.2.

In the elderly, both benign prostate conditions and prostate cancer become more common. The most common benign prostate conditions are prostatitis (inflammation of the prostate) and benign prostatic hyperplasia (BPH) (enlargement of the prostate). No evidence that prostatitis or BPH causes cancer has been found, and a man can have one or both of these disorders and develop prostate cancer as well.

A man's risk of developing prostate cancer depends on many risk factors. Age is the most common factor, because nearly 63% of cases occur in men over the age of 65. Other risk factors for prostate cancer include family history, race, and possibly diet. Men who have a father or brother with prostate cancer have a greater chance of developing prostate cancer. African American men have the highest rate of prostate cancer, while Asian and Native American men have the lowest rates. In addition, there is some evidence that a diet higher in fat, especially animal fat, may increase the risk.

In recent years, all men over the age of 50 have been advised to have a PSA test every few years. The higher his PSA level, the more likely it is that a man has prostate cancer, but there are other possible reasons for an elevated PSA reading. For example, a benign inflammation can elevate the level. If prostate cancer is present, causing a rise in the antigen in the body, the test will have a high score. A biopsy can then be done to determine whether the high score was caused by cancer or by something else.

Along with the PSA test, a physician may perform a digital rectal examination (DRE) for prostate cancer. The physician uses a gloved finger to feel the prostate gland through the rectal wall. A lumpy or hard area may be a sign of prostate cancer. Doctors often use the PSA test and DRE as prostate cancer screening tests; together, they can help doctors diagnose prostate cancer in men who have no symptoms.

Having a PSA test has seemed like a simple and useful precaution for all men, and the test is approved by the Food and Drug Administration. Because it seems like a protective measure, Medicare provides coverage for an annual PSA test for all men age 50 and older. New studies have cast doubt on whether routine screening is desirable, however. False-positive results are common when the patient has an inflammation or certain other conditions; in fact, only about 35% of positive results are due to cancer. Even if a biopsy then shows that the patient has cancer, it may be a nonaggressive, slowly growing form. Depending on the patient's age and general health, he may be likely to die from cardiovascular disease or other cause long before he would succumb to prostate cancer. In fact, in the European Randomized Study of Screening for Prostate Cancer, the researchers estimated that 1,410 men would have to be screened and 48 additional cancers would have to be detected to prevent one death from prostate cancer (Schröder et al., 2009).

A study of 1,167 Swedish men who were tested at age 60 and followed to the age of 85 indicates that the PSA test does have high predictive value (Vickers, 2010). Although few of the men having concentrations of more than 2 ng/ml (2 billionths of a gram per milliliter) develop fatal prostate cancer, 90% (78% to 100%) of deaths from prostate cancer occurred in these men. In contrast, men aged 60 having concentrations of no more than 1 ng/ml were unlikely to have clinically relevant prostate cancer. Thus, men who have a high score should be further screened, but screening may be unnecessary for others.

Even if cancer is found, the surgery may not be worth it for some patients; the chemotherapy and radiation that follow cancer surgery frequently cause incontinence and impotence, severely limiting quality of life. (The prostate gland secretes an alkaline fluid that is the largest part of a man's seminal fluid.)

Other tests for prostate cancer are being developed, and some of them may prove to be more reliable than the PSA test. Most are based on studies of a patient's ribonucleic acids or proteins. A recent study (Seppa, 2009) shows that aggressive prostate cancer cells have a higher level of the compound sarcosine than less aggressive prostate cancer cells have. Sarcosine is not found at all in healthy tissue. In time, it may be possible to determine which type of cells are in biopsied tissue of a cancer patient, so that the best treatment can be planned. Because sarcosine can be found in urine, and the PSA test relies on blood analysis, a test for identification using sarcosine would be less painful than the PSA test.

Like other procedures, the PSA test is one about which a doctor and patient should confer carefully and make an individualized decision. Risk of prostate cancer varies with age, family history, ethnicity, and other factors. If a man is at low risk, he may wish to forgo the test; if his risk is high, he may decide to have it. Men who have already had prostate cancer may need to be tested to find out whether the disease has recurred.

Hormonal therapy may be combined with radiation therapy to treat prostate cancer. If a patient has congestive heart failure as a result of coronary artery disease, hormonal therapy can increase his risk of dying (Nanda, 2009).

Skin Cancer   Skin cancer is the uncontrolled growth of abnormal skin cells. Elderly people who have been exposed to the sun for many years are at increased risk for the disease. If not controlled, skin cancer cells can spread from the skin to other tissues and organs, where the results can be serious or fatal.

There are several kinds of skin cancer, ranging from basal cell carcinoma to melanoma. Basal cell carcinoma is the most common. Melanoma is less common but more dangerous. Of all skin cancers, melanoma causes the most deaths. The stages of melanoma are shown in Table 3.3.

Symptoms of skin cancer vary greatly, and any unusual growth on the skin should be examined by a physician. The symptoms may be any of the following:

- Borders: the borders are irregular rather than round.
- Asymmetry: one half of the abnormal skin area looks unlike the other half.
- Diameter: usually (but not in every case) larger than six millimeters (diameter of a pencil eraser).
- Color: Different areas may be tan, brown, black or even white, red, or blue.
- Lack of healing: Any skin growth that bleeds or does not heal should be examined.

Table 3.2 Stages of Prostate Cancer

Stage	Diagnosis	Area Affected	Curable?
A	Found only by elevated PSA and biopsy, or during surgery for obstruction. Not palpable on digital rectal examination.	Limited to the prostate	Usually curable
B	Can be felt on rectal examination. Other tests, such as bone scans or CT/MRI scans, may be needed for diagnosis.	Limited to the prostate	Often curable
C	Determined by digital rectal exam, CT/MRI scans, and other scans	Cancer has spread beyond the prostate into local organs or tissues but has not yet metastasized or jumped to other sites	May be curable
D	Usually determined by bone scan or other studies	Cancer has spread, usually to distant lymph nodes, bones, or other sites	Not curable, but treatable

Source: American Cancer Society, 2010.

The most common form of cancer in the United States, skin cancer is found first by careful visual examination. Some doctors examine the skin using a dermatoscope, a special magnifying lens and light source that is held near the skin. Suspect growths are tested by a biopsy, and if cancer is present, surgery or other treatment can begin. Often a precancerous growth can be quickly and painlessly removed by freezing that area of the skin with liquid nitrogen.

Colorectal Cancer   Cancer may occur in any part of the large intestine. Colon cancer occurs in the longest part of the large intestine, called the colon. The last few inches of the large intestine (just inside the anus) are called the rectum. Colon and rectal cancer are sometimes discussed together, as colorectal cancer. The estimated number of deaths in 2009 from colon and rectal cancer combined was 49,920 (National Cancer Institute, 2009).

Table 3.3 Stages of Melanoma Skin Cancer

Stage	Description	Area Affected	Estimated Survival Rate*
I	The melanoma is less than 1 millimeter in thickness and may be ulcerated.	Appears limited to the skin; not found in lymph nodes or distant organs.	At least 92% of people at this stage survive 5 years or more, and at least 86% survive at least 10 more years.
II	The melanoma is from 1.01 millimeter to more than 4 millimeters thick and may be ulcerated.	Appears limited to the skin; not found in lymph nodes or distant organs.	At least 53% of people at this stage survive 5 years or more, and at least 40% survive at least 10 more years.
III	The melanoma may or may not be ulcerated. It is thick in most people.	Has spread to one to three lymph nodes, which may be enlarged, near the affected skin area. There is no distant spread.	At least 40% of people at this stage survive 5 years or more, and at least 24% survive at least 10 more years.
IV	In most cases, the melanoma is thick.	The melanoma has spread beyond the original areas to other organs or to distant parts of the skin or lymph nodes.	At least 15% of people at this stage survive 5 years or more, and at least 10% survive at least 10 more years.

*These rates may have improved in recent years and are, at best, a rough estimate of what patients can expect.
Source: National Cancer Institute, 2003.

Risk factors for colorectal cancer include the following:

- Family history of cancer of the rectum or colon
- Medical history of cancer of the rectum, colon, ovary, breast, or endometrium
- Age 50 or greater
- Medical history of colonic polyps, ulcerative colitis, or Crohn disease
- Certain hereditary conditions that affect the colon

Cancer of the colon and rectum are more common in the over-50 age group than in younger persons, and so the elderly should be screened for it, especially if they have other risk factors. Screening for this type of cancer is done with a fecal occult blood test, which is often recommended to be done annually. For this test, a small stool sample is placed on specially treated cards and sent to a laboratory for examination under a microscope. If occult (hidden) blood is found in the sample, which is an indication of possible cancer, further tests are done.

A sigmoidoscopy is an examination of the sigmoid (lower) colon and rectum. Using a flexible tube, the physician shines a light into the colon and examines it for polyps (growths). The polyps can be removed during the procedure. Some polyps are precancerous, and so their removal during the sigmoidoscopy prevents them from becoming cancerous.

A colonoscopy is similar to a sigmoidoscopy but allows the physician to examine the entire colon. Depending on the individual patient, performing a sigmoidoscopy or colonoscopy may be recommended every 5 to 10 years.

Symptoms of colorectal cancer may be manifested as a change in a person's usual bowel functions:

- Different bowel habits that persist for more than a few days
- Diarrhea or constipation
- Blood in the stool, especially if it is very dark or bright red
- Narrower stools than usual
- Frequent cramps, gas pains, fullness, or bloating
- Weight loss for unknown reasons
- Vomiting
- Fatigue

If colorectal cancer is suspected, a physician may perform a general physical examination and a digital examination of the rectum. In addition, an X-ray of the lower intestine may be done following a barium enema. (This kind of X-ray is sometimes called a lower GI series; the GI is the gastrointestinal tract.) Barium is a liquid that coats the lower GI tract, making it more visible in X-rays. Computed tomography (a CT scan) may be done, also.

Treatment depends on several factors, including the stage of the cancer (its severity and whether it has spread to other organs) and the patient's general health. Local or extensive surgery, radiation, and chemotherapy are all used for colorectal cancer. Aspirin use seems to reduce the risk of dying from colorectal cancer when it is taken by both healthy people and by those who have been diagnosed with nonmetastatic colorectal cancer (Chan et al., 2009).

Oral Cancer   Oral cancer can be found in any part of the mouth or the throat, but it usually begins in the floor of the mouth or in the tongue. Oral cancer can appear in anyone, but is more common above the age of 40, so the elderly should guard against it. In addition to age over 40, risk factors include being male, smoking (or using any tobacco products), drinking alcohol, being exposed to the sun frequently (which usually affects the lips), or having had head or neck cancer.

Oral cancer can occur in those who have lost their natural teeth. In regular checkups, a dentist will look for symptoms of oral cancer. These include loose teeth, red or white patches inside the mouth, nonhealing mouth sores, bleeding in the mouth, difficulty in swallowing, and a lump in the neck.

The risk of getting oral cancer can be lowered by avoiding tobacco products, by drinking in moderation only, and using a sunscreen-containing lip balm. As with other cancers, treatments for oral cancer can include surgery, chemotherapy, or radiation.

Dementia

As the population ages, the risk of age-related dementia in the group increases. Age-related dementias can result from circulatory dementias, the presence of Lewy bodies in brain tissue, and other causes.

One type of dementia, Alzheimer's disease, is of particular concern. Alzheimer's may appear in middle age but is more likely to be detected in those over 65. About 5% to 10% of patients develop the disease at younger ages, when it is likely to be more serious and to progress more rapidly than in elderly patients.

Maintaining good cognition is important; it increases the quality of life and prevents a future disaster for the person and their family. In recent years, there has been much enthusiasm for training the brain with cognitive tasks or computer games, but there is little research supporting this strategy. One recent study referred to in *Science* magazine (Miller, 2010) showed that people who practiced brain-training skills improved on the specific tasks but did not increase their IQs or their general cognitive ability. Instead, many psychologists suggest keeping the mind sharp by trying new skills, such as learning to play the piano, by arguing with someone with opposing political views, or by joining online discussions. These activities have intrinsic rewards regardless of whether they help the brain.

The elderly person who has no cognitive impairment is extremely rare. In typical aging, there is usually some difficulty with forgetfulness and with ability to drive, for instance. Though anyone experiencing those symptoms may worry that it is because of Alzheimer's disease, it is often the result of mild cognitive impairment, or MCI. Though MCI can be a symptom of early Alzheimer's, it may also result from stress, depression, malnutrition, lack of sleep, or other causes.

In addition to having MCI, someone who is just developing Alzheimer's disease may become disoriented in their own neighborhood, lose keys and other belongings frequently, feel confused, forget the names of family members and friends, lose the ability to express ideas, or fail to perform everyday tasks. Driving may become very difficult, and a person who does not have clinical depression may become withdrawn and lose interest in their usual activities, much as depressed people do.

Later, the disease causes more serious symptoms, so that patients cannot care for themselves and must have continual custodial care. They may suffer from delusions and become agitated. As the brain deteriorates further, it cannot control body systems that depend on neural control, and the person usually dies within 20 years of the onset of symptoms.

A variety of changes in the brain account for the symptoms of Alzheimer's. The brain of a person with Alzheimer's disease shrinks much more with age than a healthy person's would, and there is a loss of the neurotransmitter acetylcholine (the chemical that helps to send many signals across synapses to neurons that store memories). Synapses themselves disappear. Inside neurons, some cell structures become tangled, blocking the passage of chemicals and interfering with electrical signals that normally make transmission possible. A normal protein, amyloid, is converted to the abnormal beta-amyloid protein, which cannot be broken down and removed from the brain as the normal amyloid can. The abnormal beta-amyloid protein accumulates on the outsides of neurons and forms amyloid plaques (called senile plaques), further interfering with transmission of impulses in the brain. The plaques are attacked by the body's immune mechanisms that react to foreign substances. All of these changes in the brain block the transmission of impulses by sensory and motor neurons, diminishing the person's ability to sense stimuli, to think clearly, and to move normally.

One of the risk factors for Alzheimer's is genetic: The APO genes, which occur in three forms, provide the genetic code that specifies what kind of apolipoproteins a person has. Apolipoproteins in the blood carry fat and cholesterol to and from the liver. A person having two copies of the APO-Eϵ4 gene has 13 times the risk of developing Alzheimer's disease than the general population has, and someone having one copy of the APO-Eϵ4 gene has 3 to 4 times the risk that the general population has. (The general population also has APO-Eϵ2 and APO-Eϵ3 genes at the same point on a chromosome.) About 50% of Alzheimer's disease patients have the APO-Eϵ4 gene, and about 20% of the general population have it (Czech et al., 1994).

Studies are underway to determine whether identifying people who have the gene is worthwhile. Because the correlation is only 50%, and there is great worldwide geographic variation in its frequency, there may be little use in carrying out genetic studies of people who have no or few symptoms.

If there are genetic risk factors for the disease, they cannot be changed. Other unchangeable risk factors for Alzheimer's disease include being female and being elderly. Women and those over 65 are at greater risk.

Other risk factors can be controlled, however. For example, some metals (for example, arsenic, mercury, and lead) and chemical compounds (including carbon monoxide and the ingredients in tobacco) put one at great risk of brain damage. Even head injuries, depression, and sleep apnea appear to be linked to Alzheimer's disease. The same factors that lead to atherosclerosis—elevated cholesterol level, hypertension, obesity, cerebrovascular disease, diabetes, heart disease, and elevated homocysteine level—put one at risk for Alzheimer's. (Homocysteine is a protein found in the blood.) The links among cerebrovascular disease, cardiovascular disease, and Alzheimer's disease are unclear; perhaps changes in the circulatory system lead to Alzheimer's, or perhaps the disorders are separate results of one or more causes. It seems obvious, though, that controlling the substances and behaviors that lead to circulatory diseases may cut the risk of getting Alzheimer's disease.

At this time no certain way of preventing Alzheimer's disease is known. However, some studies indicate that exercising and following a Mediterranean-type diet may each help people avoid the disorder. One study (of 192 adults aged 65 or more) indicated that the diet may lower both the risk of the disease and its progression (Scarmeas et al., 2007). Another study found that three or more cups of coffee per day lowered the risk of cognitive decline in women over age 65 compared with those who drank no more than one cup of coffee per day (Ritchie et al., 2007).

The nutritional advice usually given for controlling heart disease, obesity, and diabetes applies equally to Alzheimer's disease. By eating less fat, more vegetables and fruit, and more fish, people are probably lowering their risk of cognitive decline. The fish that contain omega-3 fatty acids—salmon (including lox), tuna, sardines, and halibut—appear to have a protective effect. Fruits and vegetables that have a powerful antioxidant effect help the brain by opposing the cell damage caused by oxidation; some examples are Brussels sprouts, broccoli, collard greens, bell peppers, eggplant, spinach, blueberries, red grapes, oranges, and strawberries. Green tea, also, is an antioxidant.

Daily aerobic exercise is important for many reasons. Like nutrition, exercise affects body weight and blood levels of cholesterol and triglycerides. It probably helps protect people from Alzheimer's disease as well.

Hormone replacement therapy (HRT) is being reevaluated for its effect on cognitive function, as well as for its effect on cancer and cardiovascular disease. As with those diseases, HRT should be used with caution and on an individualized basis.

It appears that maintaining healthy levels of cholesterol and triglycerides in the blood have a protective effect against Alzheimer's disease as well as against atherosclerosis. Some experts recommend taking statins not just for lowering blood cholesterol, but also for lowering the risk of Alzheimer's disease.

If Alzheimer's is diagnosed early, the drug donepezil (Aricept) can slow down the disorder's progression. Donepezil and some other medications are ACE inhibitors; by preventing the breakdown of acetylcholine by the enzyme acetylcholinesterase, they preserve normal levels of acetylcholine. There is also a possibility that anti-inflammatory drugs such as meloxicam can protect against Alzheimer's disease along with treating circulatory disorders.

Many middle-aged and elderly people live in fear of Alzheimer's and panic at any sign of forgetfulness or confusion. Though these can be early signals of Alzheimer's disease, they can often be explained by stress or other factors. Nevertheless, if symptoms appear and do not disappear when the person gets some sleep or removes sources of stress, a doctor should be consulted. The earlier Alzheimer's is diagnosed, the more successful treatment is likely to be.

Depression

As people approach the end of life, they understandably may become sad or fearful. If these feelings continue or escalate to depression, the condition can interfere with all aspects of life.

Some symptoms of depression are the following:

- Agitation, restlessness, and irritability
- Dramatic change in appetite, often leading to weight gain or loss
- Great difficulty in concentrating
- Fatigue and loss of energy when there is no reason for it
- Feelings of hopelessness and helplessness
- Feelings of worthlessness, self-hatred, and guilt with no reason
- A loss of interest or pleasure in usual activities (such as sex or absorbing hobbies)
- Thoughts or statements about death or suicide
- Insomnia or excessive sleeping

It is important for physicians and caregivers to screen patients for depression by using a quick assessment tool such as the Geriatric Depression Scale (Poon, 1986b; a short form is shown in Appendix A), or by simply asking whether they feel depressed, and to treat them if necessary. Even the terminally ill can have a better quality of life if they are not depressed.

The exogenous (externally caused) depression seen in many of the elderly is a result of circumstances (boredom with life in a nursing home, neglect by children, failing physical health, and so on), and is distinct from the endogenous (clinical) depression that may occur in people of any age, even in children. (Clinical depression is found in about 1% to 2% of the elderly population, according to Barry et al. [2008]).The exact causes of clinical depression are unknown. The disorder may be partly hereditary and may be biochemical as well as psychological.

For older women, more than for older men, symptoms of depression are likely to appear; in addition, their depression is apt to last longer (Barry et al., 2008). From 1998 through 2005, a group of 754 men and women aged 70 or more self-reported every 18 months about symptoms of major depression. Thirty-six percent of the respondents became depressed at some time during the study; nearly half of them continued to be depressed for three years thereafter, and almost 5% were depressed for the remainder of the study. At each checkpoint, more women than men were depressed, and their depression lasted longer. In contrast, men were more likely than women to die while they were depressed. The researchers stated that future studies should focus on whether elderly women need to be treated more aggressively for depression or whether they are less likely to respond to conventional treatments for the disorder.

A mildly depressed old person may respond to mood-lifting measures such as exercise, but these measures are unlikely to help sufferers from true clinical depression, which is usually treated with psychotherapy or antidepressant drugs. Antidepressant drugs include the following:

- Selective serotonin reuptake inhibitors. These are the most commonly used antidepressants. The drugs include fluoxetine (Prozac), sertraline (Zoloft), paroxetine (Paxil), fluvoxamine (Luvox), citalopram (Celexa), and escitalopram (Lexapro).
- Serotonin norepinephrine reuptake inhibitors (SNRIs). These are also commonly used for depression. Some are desvenlafaxine (Pristiq), venlafaxine (Effexor), and duloxetine (Cymbalta).
- Other medicines used to treat depression are tricyclic antidepressants, bupropion (Wellbutrin), and monoamine oxidase inhibitors.

People who have psychotic symptoms, such as delusions or hallucinations, may need antipsychotic medications instead of, or in addition to, antidepressants.

Antidepressants are often prescribed for people with exogenous depression as well. Whether they are overprescribed is a controversial topic among practitioners; some critics believe that psychotherapy and attention to diet and exercise are more appropriate for mildly depressed people.

Clinical depression can lead to suicide. Anyone who has thoughts of suicide, thoughts of harming themselves or others, or other suicide warning signs should seek help. They can call 911 or a suicide hotline or go to a nearby emergency room. Telephone numbers to call from anywhere in the United States, 24 hours a day, 7 days a week, are 1-800-SUICIDE or 1-800-999-9999.

Diabetes

According to the American Diabetes Association (2010), about 23.6 million Americans have diabetes. The disease occurs in two forms: Type 1 and Type 2. Type 1 is much more severe, but both types can greatly damage health. Type 1 diabetes, also called juvenile diabetes, primarily strikes people when they are still young. However, it lasts for a lifetime and exacts its greatest toll on the elderly. People with type 1 diabetes cannot make any insulin—the hormone that enables liver, muscle, and fat tissue cells to take up and use glucose from the blood—and so the victims must take insulin injections, limit their intake of calories and carbohydrates, and get regular exercise. Typically, a person with this disorder must use a lance to draw blood and measure the glucose level in it several times a day, which takes time and is somewhat painful. Keeping the blood sugar level within a certain range, neither too high (hyperglycemia) or too low (hypoglycemia), is essential. If the disease is uncontrolled, it can lead to kidney damage, blindness, and other serious effects. Dialysis may be needed if the kidneys do not function normally.

Type 2 diabetes, also called adult-onset diabetes, is common in many elderly people and in obese people of any age (National Institutes of Health, 2008). The Islets of Langerhans, cells imbedded in the pancreas, make too little insulin in people with this disease. Type 2 diabetes is often associated with heart disease as well as obesity. A strict diet and exercise can help control the disease, and some patients are helped by oral medications that stimulate insulin production. As the disease worsens, insulin injections may be needed. In end-stage renal disease, which can result from either type of diabetes, the kidneys have been damaged so much that frequent dialysis is needed to rid the body of toxins.

Because of the obesity epidemic in the United States and many other countries, type 2 diabetes is becoming more common. Some experts have estimated that, by the year 2020, half of the population will be obese. However, a recent report claims that the gain in obesity has leveled off (Flegal, 2010). Even so, already a great number of people are overweight or obese and thus in danger of getting diabetes and other disorders.

Either type of diabetes can decrease blood flow to the feet. Neuropathy (degeneration of the nerves) is a complication of the decreased blood flow. Some diabetic patients with that condition cannot feel heat that can burn their skin, or they experience tingling or other sensations. In severe cases, the lack of circulation leads to tissue damage and gangrene, and part of a limb must be amputated.

Erectile Dysfunction

As advertising has made everyone realize, erectile dysfunction (ED) is common in aging men. There is no single cause of erectile dysfunction. In some cases, an underlying condition such as obesity or diabetes causes ED. Or a hormonal imbalance or a muscle or circulatory disorder may lead to erectile dysfunction. Treating the condition can cure ED at the same time. The underlying problem can be physical or psychological; for example, someone who is under stress at work or anxious about a marital partner can develop ED even if there is no physical condition causing it. Fatigue and depression are other psychological causes of erectile dysfunction.

Usually, there is a physical cause for ED (Mayo Clinic, 2010a). Some of the physical causes include:

- Atherosclerosis
- Hypertension
- Heart disease
- Multiple sclerosis
- Obesity
- Diabetes (type 1 or type 2)
- Parkinson's disease
- Metabolic syndrome
- Low testosterone level
- Peyronie's disease
- Use of tobacco
- Abuse of alcohol or drugs

- Treatments for prostate cancer or enlarged prostate
- Injury to the pelvic area or spinal cord

ED is treated in various ways. Oral drugs act by enhancing effects of the body's natural nitric oxide; the penis muscles relax, blood flow increases, and an erection is possible. These drugs include sildenafil (Viagra), tadalafil (Cialis), and vardenafil (Levitra). There are also some over-the-counter supplements and herbal remedies for erectile dysfunction, but they should be used only if approved by a physician. ED drugs are safe and effective for some men but dangerous for others. A patient may need to try different drugs and dosages under a physician's guidance to find the best one for him, and the physician should also be aware of all other drugs being taken. If the patient takes nitrate drugs (such as nitroglycerine) for angina, blood-thinning drugs, or drugs for hypertension, he should not take a drug for erectile dysfunction without a physician's direction. Similarly, heart disease, stroke, diabetes, or very high or low blood pressure are usually contraindications for ED drug treatment.

In addition to these oral medications, erectile dysfunction can be treated with injections. The patient can inject alprostadil into the base or side of his penis to produce an erection that lasts about an hour. Or, an alprostadil suppository can be placed inside the penis. If he has a low level of testosterone, he may benefit from replacement therapy with the hormone.

In some cases, medications are ineffective or contraindicated for an individual patient, but other aids are available. He may be able to use a penis pump, which is a vacuum constriction device that pulls blood into the penis long enough for him to sustain an erection. Surgical penile implants of silicone or polyurethane rods are used for some patients, or blood vessel surgery may be needed.

Falls

Young people can recover easily from most tumbles, but in the elderly, falls can be dangerous or fatal. Breaking a hip, especially, is likely to be followed by a patient's final ride to a hospital. Being aware of the causes and prevention of falls is vital for older people and their caregivers.

In some cases, a fall is caused by a preexisting physical condition. Even a brief drop in blood pressure can lead to a bad fall. (Postural hypotension is a drop in blood pressure that occurs when a person sits or stands suddenly.) In a study of 336 people aged 75 or more (Tinetti et al., 1988) that was reported in the *New England Journal of Medicine,* researchers found that other conditions increasing the risk of falls included the use of sedatives, the use of at least four prescription medicines, impaired limb strength or range of motion, poor balance, impaired skills in transferring (from a bed to a chair, for example), and impaired gait.

In drop attacks, the legs of the patient, usually an elderly person, go out from under them, and they fall to the floor without losing consciousness. This may not cause harm if the floor is soft, but it is a signal that the person should be examined by a doctor to determine the cause.

Falls can result from a person's cardiovascular condition. Some people may experience intermittent cardiac arrhythmia, for instance. It can be precipitated by various factors, such as lowered oxygen level at high altitudes, apnea, chronic renal failure, certain foods, or alcohol. It may be accompanied by dizziness, chest pain, or fainting. Arrhythmias can be controlled with lidocaine or other drugs. Fainting (syncope) results when too little oxygen-carrying blood reaches the brain. Some fainting is due to a vasovagal attack, the action of a vagus nerve on the heart or blood vessels.

Both as symptoms of illness and as causes of damage to the body, falls must not be ignored. In the Tinetti et al. study, during one year, 108 (32%) of the people studied fell at least once, 24% of those who fell had serious injuries, and 6% had fractures.

Some falls can be prevented by creating a safer home environment. The bathroom is a dangerous room in this respect, and the floor should be unwaxed and uncluttered with throw rugs. Even for younger people, grab bars near the tub and shower can prevent a fall. For anyone who has trouble standing, grab bars next to the toilet are useful. Bright lighting is also important.

If stairs are many and steep, a stair lift can make getting up and down the stairs possible. Even without a stair lift, stairs can be made safer for the elderly: Handrails on both sides help a person stay balanced and to climb or descend slowly. There should always be proper lighting, so that someone with poor vision does not fail to see the bottom step. This can be provided with easily reachable light switches at the bottom and top of the stairs or with motion-sensitive lights that go off automatically to save electricity. On painted or varnished stairs, nonslip material such as that used on boats can provide a safer surface.

Hearing Disorders

When vibrations in the air reach the ear, they are transferred through the outer and middle ear to the inner ear, which is connected to the part of the brain that interprets impulses as sounds. In the inner ear, the vibrations pass through fluid in the cochlea, which is a snail-shaped structure. Hairs in the cochlea are set in motion by the vibrations and send electrical signals to the brain through a nerve.

Loss of hearing is very common in the elderly, and hearing aids are not covered by Medicare. Thus, many elderly people deny their increasing deafness and postpone being tested by an audiologist. Eventually, hearing loss reaches the point where the person must admit the problem or become more and more isolated from others. (In fact, some of the very old who are afflicted with both deafness and blindness say that deafness is much worse as a cause of social isolation.)

In adults, deafness can result from drugs that affect the ears or the brain and from trauma, loud noises, illness, infections, or tumors. A gradual buildup of earwax also can interfere significantly with hearing. Because deafness is caused by changes in both the ears and the brain, the remedies for the condition vary in different individuals. Hearing aids help some people greatly but make little difference to others. An audiologist can help determine the source of hearing loss and refer the patient to a hearing aid specialist.

During a routine physical exam, a physician will probably examine the ears with a lighted instrument called an otoscope. Examination with an otoscope can uncover obstruction by objects or earwax in the ear canal, injury to the ear, and evidence of infection.

An audiologist will go farther, carrying out an audiologic evaluation of hearing. This may consist of a variety of tests, including a tuning fork test, a whisper test, tests with earphones, and speech reception tests. Also, the audiologist will determine whether sounds travel into the inner ear or are merely bounced back from the tympanum (eardrum) and the middle-ear bones (the hammer, anvil, and stirrup). A test of otoacoustic emissions measures the response to different sounds (such as a click or tone) by the inner ear.

Some have speculated that deafness is increasing in the population because the baby boomers and younger people have been exposed to extremely loud popular music since the 1960s. President Bill Clinton did his generation a great service by admitting he could not hear and by getting a hearing aid, which lessened the stigma of deafness.

Nearly all older people have some presbycusis (high-frequency hearing loss). As a result, they have trouble in discriminating some sounds, especially when there is background noise—in a noisy restaurant or at a party, for example. Tinnitus (ringing or roaring in the ears) also may interfere with hearing. It results from some disorders and some drugs.

There is a wide variety of hearing aids; some fit behind the ear, some in the ear canal. They may be either quite visible or invisible. In recent years, many hearing aids have been developed that are programmable by the audiologist or by the wearer. Prices range widely, from a few hundred to thousands of dollars. Because many insurance plans do not cover hearing aids, the patient should choose carefully and consult several sources before deciding on one type. In general, it is preferable to avoid free hearing tests and sellers who offer only one brand of hearing aid.

Even without a hearing aid, deaf persons can make behavioral changes that help them hear better. It is helpful to face someone who is speaking and to focus on the speaker's lips, for example. If possible, noisy restaurants and other environments that interfere with hearing can be avoided. Friends and family can help considerably by speaking more slowly and a little more loudly—without shouting—and enunciating.

Heart Attacks

Like strokes, heart attacks are most often caused by thrombi (blood clots) blocking the blood vessels. A blood clot can block the arteries to the heart or brain. If the coronary arteries (arteries on the heart) are blocked, too little oxygen is delivered to the heart muscle by the blood, and a myocardial infarction (heart attack) results.

The symptoms of a heart attack are not limited to chest pain. Any of the following may be heart attack symptoms:

- Chest discomfort (such as feelings of crushing or squeezing)
- Sweating
- Weakness or tiredness
- Lightheadedness
- Nausea or vomiting
- Shortness of breath
- Anxiety

For both sexes, chest pain is the most common sign that a heart attack is imminent, but women are more likely to experience atypical symptoms as well. In a National Institutes of Health study of 515 women heart patients, researchers found that 70% had sudden, severe fatigue in the weeks preceding their attacks, and smaller percentages had other symptoms, such as sleep disturbances. Because atypical symptoms may not be treated in emergency rooms with the same seriousness as chest pain, a woman who thinks she is having a heart attack may need to be assertive about being tested (Women's Heart Foundation, 2010).

Heart attacks are treated with thrombolytic (blood-clot dissolving) drugs, usually tissue plasminogen activator. Other drugs are sometimes used; they include lanoteplase, staphylokinase, tenecteplase, and streptokinase.

Thrombolytic medicines can quickly break down even a major clot, reopening the blood vessel. This can allow blood to begin flowing to the heart. The treatment with a thrombolytic drug should begin within 12 hours of a heart attack's onset. The American Heart Association recommends that thrombolysis begin within 90 minutes of arrival at an emergency room.

Whether thrombolytic medication is prescribed depends on several factors. These include the patient's age and gender, history of chest pain, previous or current damage to the heart, heart rate and rhythm, the size and position of the auricles and ventricles in the heart, and any drugs or devices (such as a pacemaker) being used to regulate the heart. The heart rate and rhythm are measured with an electrocardiogram. If the patient has bleeding problems (such as bleeding ulcers), has a recent head injury or trauma, has just had surgery, has uncontrolled hypertension, or is pregnant, thrombolytic drugs probably will not be administered.

In most cases, tissue plasminogen activator restores some blood flow to the heart muscle, but the blood flow may be abnormal, and there may be some damage to the heart. Additional therapy, usually surgical, may be required.

Hypertension

Hypertension is important less for itself than for the disorders it causes. It may lead to cardiac effects—myocardial infarction, cardiac failure, angina, and left ventricular hypertrophy—or to damage to the brain, kidneys, and other organs. People who have hypertension may experience headaches, diarrhea, and other symptoms that should not be ignored.

Infections

Elderly patients are especially vulnerable to hospital-acquired infections, both because they are more apt than younger persons to be hospitalized for other reasons and because they have less ability to fight off infection. One infection that has risen in the elderly is infective endocarditis, an infection of the tissue lining the heart. Although it is most likely to affect the heart's valves, it can attack shunts, catheters, and pacemakers—all found in many elderly patients (Akpunoni et al., 2008).

Pneumonia in the elderly was once a common cause of death. Today cardiovascular disease is more likely to kill an elderly person, because antibiotics are available for pneumonia caused by bacteria, usually *Streptococcus pneumoniae*. Treatment with antibiotics cures patients whose pneumonia was caused by antibiotic-susceptible bacteria. (Viral pneumonia, on the other hand, cannot be cured by antibiotics.) Nevertheless, pneumonia remains a danger for those who may have other debilitating diseases and for those who may be frail in general. It is a familiar disease in nursing homes.

Symptoms of pneumonia may be limited to delirium in some elderly patients (Marrie, 2000), making it more difficult to diagnose. In other elderly patients, the usual expected symptoms of coughing, fever, chest pain, difficulty in breathing, and so on are obvious.

Risk is greater for patients aged 70 or more, those who suffer from asthma, and those who are alcoholics. Other risk factors include being a man, being a debilitated patient in a nursing home, having incontinence, and being unable to take oral medicines.

At least one vaccination for pneumonia with the Pneumovax vaccine is needed by the elderly and by younger people with some diseases, but it may be resisted by some patients (because it causes a more painful reaction than influenza vaccines do), and it may be inadvisable for others. Recommendations have changed over the years, but a repeated vaccination after 5 or 10 years may be advised for anyone over 65.

Anyone who has had chickenpox can get the painful skin rash known as shingles (or herpes zoster). The virus that causes chickenpox in childhood can lie dormant in the body and reappear many years afterward to cause shingles. The elderly are especially at risk; shingles is more common in those aged 50 and older. In addition to causing extreme pain, shingles can bring about headache, fever, chills, and an upset stomach. In very rare cases, it can cause more severe symptoms, such as blindness, or even be fatal.

In 2006, Zostavax, a vaccine for shingles, appeared. It prevented shingles in about half the over-60 people participating in clinical trials. It also reduced pain in some of those who did get shingles. The Centers for Disease Control and Prevention recommends that adults over the age of 60 receive a single dose of the vaccine. In some cases, however, people should avoid the vaccine. A history of allergies to any component of the vaccine (including gelatin, neomycin, and other compounds) is one danger signal. Also, anyone with a weakened immune system or with active, untreated tuberculosis should not have the shingles vaccine. Mild illnesses mean vaccination should be postponed until the person is well.

Mild reactions to the vaccine, similar to those that occur with the influenza vaccine, are common. No serious reactions have been reported. If an allergic reaction does occur (causing symptoms such as difficulty breathing, hives, or dizziness), the person should seek medical help immediately. Insurance coverage for the shingles vaccine varies, but for those with Medicare Part D, the cost can be as low as $39—a small price for important protection.

Menopause

Some women reach the end of their childbearing years with no symptoms, but many have the hot flashes (sudden, uncontrollable waves of heat), sweating, and other uncomfortable and embarrassing problems associated with menopause. The symptoms result from hormonal imbalance, when less estrogen is produced by the body. Few effective remedies are available, aside from drinking quantities of cold water that lead to increased urination without completely relieving the menopausal symptoms.

Hormone replacement therapy, or HRT (which includes estrogen), was the standard treatment for decades as a treatment for the hot flashes, vaginal dryness, and other menopausal symptoms that affect a woman's quality of life. In addition, estrogen reduces the risk of colon cancer and hip fractures. Altogether, it appeared to be a fountain of youth for aging women. However, HRT has caused enormous concern among women and their physicians in recent years.

In 1982, the National Institutes of Health began the Women's Health Initiative (WHI), the largest clinical trial ever conducted. The hormone preparation tested was Prempro, which contains both estrogen and progesterone. The study was canceled suddenly in 2002, when it showed that there was a slight increase in heart attacks, strokes, blood clots in lungs, and breast cancer among 10,000 healthy postmenopausal women using Prempro for one year. In another study—an analysis of 121,000 women's responses to a questionnaire from the Nurses' Health Study—researchers also found that estrogen (alone or with progesterone) increased the risk of stroke in both younger and older women (Grodstein et al., 2008).

Though many women stopped taking HRT after the 2002 results were announced, some experts still feel that it is useful for the first five years of menopause in women who lack risk factors such as a family history of heart disease or breast cancer. That recommendation is based in part on a second WHI study (Stefanick et al., 2006). In contrast to earlier findings, the second study found that "treatment with CEE [conjugated equine estrogens] alone for 7.1 years does not increase breast cancer incidence in postmenopausal women with prior hysterectomy and may decrease the risk of early stage disease and ductal carcinomas." The adverse effects reported in the first study may have been brought about by the addition of progesterone to estrogen. The second study did show that women taking estrogen alone were more likely to have abnormalities in their breasts and to need follow-up after mammography screening than women taking a placebo. (No results were reported for cardiovascular effects.) The authors recommended that use of CEE be based on consideration of the individual woman's potential risks and benefits. Obviously, many factors are involved in the decision of whether to use HRT, and physicians and patients should consider them carefully. Abstracts of the two WHI studies are in Appendix A.

Musculoskeletal Disorders

Arthritis   Osteoarthritis (which is also known as degenerative arthritis) results when bony surfaces in the joints are worn and new bone grows laterally. The spurs seen on X-rays are new bone growth. Osteoarthritis is often associated with a prior injury to a joint, even if it occurred in childhood.

All adults past the age of 40 have osteoarthritis that can be seen in X-rays of the cervical (neck) spine. With further aging, arthritis affects the weight-bearing joints, such as the knees and ankles.

Weight control and exercise are the measures most often prescribed for osteoarthritis. The pain of milder osteoarthritis can be alleviated by taking nonsteroidal anti-inflammatory drugs (NSAIDs). In severe cases, joint replacement is often successful (Gibson, 2008).

Rheumatoid arthritis is an autoimmune disorder that is much more severe than osteoarthritis. In general, rheumatoid arthritis begins in middle age and progresses in later years, but in some cases it strikes elderly people suddenly. The joints are swollen and tender; they may become greatly deformed in time. Other symptoms, such as anorexia and fever, may accompany the obvious physical signs.

There is no real cure for rheumatoid arthritis, but the disease process can be slowed, and mortality lessened, by methotrexate and other drugs (Merck Manual of Geriatrics, 2010). NSAIDs are prescribed for the pain. Therapy should begin early in order to protect the joints from breakdown and prevent disability.

Osteoporosis   A fragile skeleton can be damaged easily by a fall, or it may spontaneously break. In fact, the lifetime risk from hip, forearm, and vertebral fractures in white men is about 40%; this is comparable to the risk for cardiovascular disease.

It is obvious that preventing the development of osteoporosis is extremely important for the elderly. Less apparently, the prevention should begin early. Today teenagers drink too little milk, increasing their danger of the disease later in life. Drinking milk and eating calcium-rich foods are useful in prevention. Vitamin D_3 also is important and is often lacking in people who are exposed to little sunlight. (Getting some sun on bare skin for about 10 to 15 minutes a day twice a week is enough to stimulate the body to produce the vitamin). Lack of exercise, especially weight-bearing exercise, contributes to the disease's development.

Millions of Americans, especially white and Asian women, have osteoporosis. Some risk factors for the disease include:

- Broken bones during adulthood
- Family history
- Premenopausal ovariectomy
- Early menopause
- Extended bed rest
- Too little calcium in the diet throughout life
- Medications that affect the bones
- Small body frame

Men, too, may have osteoporosis, especially as they age. According to the National Osteoporosis Foundation (National Osteoporosis Foundation, 2011), 12 million men in the United States have low bone mass that puts them at risk for osteoporosis, and 2 million men already have the disorder. After the age of 50, 25% of men are at risk of breaking a bone because of osteoporosis. Though hip fractures are very serious for anyone, men are more likely than women to die in the first year following a hip fracture.

Osteopenia is an early stage of osteoporosis that is a strong danger signal. Bone loss has started, but osteoporosis can be postponed or avoided if the person begins changing diet and exercise habits and takes medication.

Free or low-cost bone-density tests are widely available. These give some indication of a person's status, but many physicians suggest the more informative DEXA-scan (dual-energy X-ray absorptiometry scan) for patients who are over 65 or are at risk for osteoporosis. (This scan may not be covered by Medicare or other insurance.) The scan provides information about the patient's risk for a fracture (broken bone).

In some of the elderly, a vitamin D deficiency—resulting from too little of the vitamin in the diet or from too little exposure to sunlight—can lead to an increase in osteoclast activity. Many physicians and orthopedists (bone specialists) are beginning to prescribe large doses of vitamin D for their elderly patients who are deficient in the vitamin. Although the vitamin can be toxic if taken in excess, the toxic dosage is extremely high and is not likely to be exceeded.

Other measures that can help decrease the loss of bone mass are not smoking and limiting alcohol consumption. Because some medicines—glucocorticoids, some cancer drugs, some sleeping pills, and others—can lead to bone loss, they should be used with caution.

Various drugs are available for the treatment of osteoporosis. They include raloxifene, which is a selective estrogen receptor modulator; calcitonin, a hormone that increases bone mass in the spine; biphosphonates, which slow the breakdown of bone; estrogen, which increases bone mass in the spine and hips; and parathyroid hormone, which increases bone density in the spine and hips. Anyone who has osteoporosis must be extremely careful not to fall and to take precautions that lower the likelihood of falling.

Therapy for osteoporosis includes exercise, such as walking and tai chi (which also improves balance). Drugs that contribute to bone mineralization, such as alendronate, estrogen, calcium, vitamin D_3, and calcitonin, are prescribed. Some specialists prescribe parathyroid hormone for patients with low levels of it. For those who have already had fractures, patients and their families need to inspect their homes to remove any loose rugs, dangling cords, or other items that may lead to falls. A cane or walker increases confidence and encourages the patient to walk more.

Parkinson's Disease

Brain cells produce a substance called dopamine, which facilitates transmission of neural impulses between cells. In motor system disorders, there is a loss of the cells that make dopamine, and so the brain cannot send messages to the neurons that control muscle movements. Parkinson's disease is one kind of motor system disorder. It is chronic, and the symptoms become worse over time. No chemical tests for Parkinson's are available; the diagnosis is based on neurological exams and observations of the patient's symptoms.

Parkinson's disease is diagnosed mainly by its symptoms, which include tremor in the arms, legs, and face; rigidity of movement; bradykinesia (slow movement); and difficulty in coordination and balance. The symptoms may begin early and grow worse over time, becoming more evident in the elderly. The severity varies among individuals. Eventually the disease can interfere with simple activities such as swallowing food, speaking, and sleeping.

Although no cure exists, many medications help to control the symptoms. Levodopa and cardidopa are usually prescribed together; brain cells convert the levodopa to dopamine, and the conversion is delayed by the cardidopa until the levodopa reaches the brain. Rigidity and bradykinesia are usually controlled best by these drugs, and other drugs may help to control other symptoms, such as imbalance. For patients who do not respond to the drugs, surgery or deep-brain electrical stimulation may help (National Institute of Neurological Disorders and Stroke, 2010b). It is hoped that stem-cell research can lead to a cure for this disease.

Often an elderly person has a tremor that appears to be caused by Parkinson's disease (and may be misdiagnosed as Parkinson's) but is actually a less serious disorder, essential tremor. Unlike Parkinson's, essential tremor does not respond to the drugs used for Parkinson's; increases if the affected body part is moved; and lessens if the patient ingests alcohol, barbiturates, or beta blockers. In addition, patients do not have the bradykinesia, imbalance, rigidity, and impaired gait found in Parkinson's patients.

Sleep Disorders

Sleep is essential for health at all ages. As Shakespeare's Macbeth said in despair, sleep "knits up the raveled sleave of care," restoring mental equilibrium as well as physical health.

In the elderly, illness or other factors may interfere with getting a good night's sleep. As people age, they tend to go to bed earlier and rise earlier than when they were younger. However, insomnia keeps many from falling asleep or may cause them to wake in the middle of the night, then toss and turn for hours. Some of the elderly wake up extremely early and are unable to go back to sleep. Worrying about problems may cause sleeplessness. In addition, age affects the type of sleep they have. The deepest sleep is called non-REM (rapid eye movement). The elderly tend to spend less time in non-REM sleep and more time in REM sleep, when there is more dreaming.

However insomnia affects people, it can leave them tired and irritable. They may find it hard to think clearly, may feel depressed, and even may be more likely to have falls and accidents if they are not well rested.

Over-the-counter or prescription sleep medicines may help, but they are a temporary aid for insomnia. Developing good sleep habits and treating physical or emotional problems that may affect sleep can lead to a permanent improvement.

Sleep habits that can help include the following recommendations:

- Provide a safe, restful environment for sleeping. Lock the doors and windows of the home, have a telephone and lamp within easy reach of the bed, and turn on nightlights in the hallways and bathroom.
- Never smoke in bed. If a heating pad is used in bed, be sure it is turned off before you fall asleep, because it may burn.
- Make the bedroom conducive to sleep. Don't watch television there or read thrillers in bed. Have a pillow that supports your head and neck properly and enough blankets in cold weather.
- Do not eat large meals or drink caffeinated beverages in the evening. Drinking alcohol may cause you to wake up during the night, even if it seems to help you fall asleep. Drink less liquid of any type during the evening if it makes you get up to use the bathroom at night.

- Exercise during the day, not within three hours of bedtime. Try not to nap during the day if you have trouble sleeping at night.
- In daytime, get out in the sunlight.
- At bedtime, do anything nontoxic that you know will help you sleep: Drink a little milk, make a to-do list for the next day so that you will not lie awake thinking about things you need to do, or do whatever else you find effective.

For many people, these measures will help greatly. Some conditions, however, cause sleep disturbances that call for more extreme measures. If a medication is causing insomnia, it may be possible to substitute another drug for it, for instance. Some disorders that interfere with sleep can be cured or alleviated. Anti-anxiety drugs are useful for some people.

One sleep-disturbing condition is apnea. The apnea sufferer stops breathing periodically during sleep, gasping for air and snoring loudly. Surprisingly, the person may not realize he or she is not breathing properly, but may have to be told about it by a bed partner who is kept awake. During the day, apnea causes sleepiness. Sleep apnea may seem more irritating than dangerous, but it is a serious condition. Left untreated, it can cause hypertension, stroke, or loss of memory.

Specialists in sleep problems can diagnose sleep apnea and treat it. The standard treatment includes a device called continuous positive air pressure (CPAP), which pushes air into the lungs during the sleep, bringing about normal breathing and sleeping. Other treatments may use dental devices or surgery.

A new and less obtrusive method of treating sleep apnea is based on exercises used in speech therapy (Guimarães et al., 2009). In a small controlled study, patients with apnea were treated with exercises for the tongue, soft palate, and pharynx. Their snoring, daytime sleepiness, and other symptoms decreased; in addition, their neck circumference decreased. Thinner necks are associated with less occurrence of apnea.

Other conditions that can cause sleep disorders are restless legs syndrome and periodic limb movement disorder. With restless legs syndrome, which tends to be worse at night, people feel sensations in their legs such as tingling, pins and needles, or crawling. Periodic limb movement disorder makes people jerk and kick their legs often during sleep. Medications for both conditions can be prescribed.

Alzheimer's patients may sleep too much or too little and may wander about the house. Their caregivers, who often miss sleep themselves as a result, need to protect the patients by making sure they cannot fall down stairs, slip on loose rugs, or fall in the bathroom during the night.

Stroke

People of all ages, but especially the elderly, should know the signs of a stroke. Immediate treatment can help many stroke victims, but it must not be delayed. The signs are:

- Sudden numbness or weakness of the face, arm, or leg, especially on one side
- Sudden confusion or trouble speaking
- Sudden trouble with walking, dizziness, or loss of balance
- Sudden trouble with vision in one or both eyes
- Severe headache without a known cause

To determine the type of stroke to be treated, a doctor will perform tests such as a CT scan. Some strokes are caused by clots in the bloodstream, others by hemorrhaging of blood vessels in the brain. The treatments for the two types are very different: For the first type, thrombolytic (clot-dissolving) medicines are given; for the second, bleeding must be controlled. The wrong type of treatment can be dangerous, even fatal. If the stroke has been caused by a hemorrhage, thrombolytics can increase the bleeding. If the stroke was caused by a clot, however, giving clot-dissolving medicines within three hours of the first stroke symptoms can limit brain damage and disability.

To decide whether to use clot-dissolving medicines, the attending physician will order a CT scan of the patient's brain to be sure there is no bleeding. In addition, the physician will take a medical history and order a physical examination showing a significant stroke.

Sometimes the symptoms of a stroke appear but disappear within an hour. In that case, a transient ischemic attack (TIA) has occurred. A TIA is a very brief stroke. As in any stroke, the victim of a TIA may be confused, feel numbness or weakness, or slur his or her speech. A TIA is less serious than an acute stroke, but until a diagnosis is made, it should be treated as an acute stroke.

Often TIAs are early warnings that people will have acute strokes later on. Thus, anyone who has had a TIA should take steps to avoid strokes, such as losing weight, taking drugs as needed to control hypertension, and not smoking.

Urinary Incontinence

Nocturia, or nighttime urination, is common in people over the age of 65. Urinary incontinence may also be a problem in daytime.

Incontinence may be a temporary condition caused by drugs such as diuretics, narcotics, antipsychotic medications, sleeping pills or muscle relaxants, antihistamines, antidepressants, or calcium channel blockers. If the drugs are discontinued or the dosage lowered, incontinence may no longer be a problem. Other temporary conditions that can lead to incontinence are infections in the urinary tract or vagina and severe constipation. In these cases, the incontinence can be a useful symptom that signals a (usually treatable) disorder.

In elderly people, incontinence falls into the general categories of urge incontinence, stress incontinence, overflow incontinence, and functional incontinence (Mayo Clinic, 2010b).

Urge incontinence is the frequent, sudden urge to urinate; it is the most common type in the elderly. The person has little control of the bladder and may urinate while drinking, sleeping, or hearing water running. They may need to urinate more than seven times daily or more than twice nightly. It is also known as spastic bladder, overactive bladder, or reflex incontinence.

Stress incontinence is often seen in elderly women, especially those who have borne children earlier in life. It results from weakened pelvic muscles, damaged neural control of the bladder, or other anatomic age-related conditions. The bladder tends to leak urine when the person sneezes or puts pressure on the pelvic muscles in some other way.

Overflow incontinence is caused by weakened bladder muscles. As a result, the bladder cannot be completely emptied, and so the patient urinates very frequently, dribbles urine constantly, or both. People with this disorder may have nerve damage, an enlarged prostate, or blockage of the urethra.

Elderly people who have Parkinson's disease, Alzheimer's disease, or arthritis may have functional incontinence. They cannot reach a bathroom soon enough because they either cannot move quickly or do not realize they need to urinate.

Although failure to control urination may seem like a trivial problem and may even be the subject of jokes, it can become a major issue for its victims. Fear of having an accident causes some to stay at home when they could be visiting friends, doing paid or volunteer work, or going to plays and concerts. That, in turn, can lead to getting fewer invitations to go out. The incontinent person can become increasingly isolated from needed social interactions. Still, out of embarrassment or lack of information, they may fail to seek help from physicians.

Also, physicians in general practice may not be well prepared to treat their patients for incontinence. In one study carried out in Germany (Wiedemann and Füsgen, 2009), for example, researchers found that only 35% of general practitioners had studied the treatment of incontinence in medical school. Most of their training in the subject had been gained at conferences.

Of the physicians questioned, 76.6% referred their incontinent patients to specialists.

In most cases, however, the condition can be alleviated, and the suffering is unnecessary. Measures such as drinking plenty of water, which is counterintuitive but effective; losing weight; avoiding caffeine; and doing tai chi chih, Kegel, or other exercises that strengthen the pelvic muscles all help. Drugs that control urination, such as oxybutynin, are available from physicians, and some hospitals offer helpful classes. In some cases, surgery is needed.

Visual Disorders

Many visual problems arise or become worse as people age. Some can be alleviated with simple alterations in surroundings; others can improve with the use of eyeglasses or other measures.

Environmental changes that can aid many people include proper lighting (bright enough without causing glare), large-print books and magazines, nonprescription reading glasses, hand lenses, audio books, and large-print settings on computers. To compensate for poor vision, it is helpful to put colored tape on stair edges, purchase items such as cell phones and calculators that have large numbered keys, and add large-print labels to appliances or tools. Wide-brimmed hats and sunglasses protect the eyes from glare.

Some Web sites contain special features that make them easier to use by the visually impaired. For example, the National Institute on Aging and the National Library of Medicine provide the site www.nihseniorhealth.gov; the text can be read aloud to the viewer, or the type can be made larger.

Vision in general tends to decline with aging, and by the age of 80, more than half of Americans either have cataracts or have had cataract surgery. Cataracts are most common in the elderly, but they may also result from diabetes, prolonged exposure to sunlight, overuse of alcohol, or smoking. They may be postponed by wearing a broad-brimmed hat and sunglasses, by not smoking, and by good nutrition (including green vegetables and other sources of antioxidants).

Cataracts develop in the lens of the eye, the clear portion through which light is focused on the retina. Proteins in the lens clump together to form cataracts, so light cannot pass through the lens easily. As a result, too little light reaches the retina, and vision is decreased. As cataracts continue to develop, the person's color vision is affected. The lens itself becomes brown or yellow, and colors are perceived incorrectly. Over time, the field of vision becomes increasingly blurred and discolored.

Cataracts usually begin to develop during middle age, affecting vision gradually. Most people reach the point of needing surgery during their 60s. Cataract surgery is fairly simple and, in more than 90% of cases, results in improved vision. It is covered by Medicare.

People in their 60s and older should have an eye examination at least every two years. The pupils must be dilated so the ophthalmologist can see into the eye clearly. Cataracts and other vision disorders, such as age-related macular degeneration and glaucoma, can be discovered during the examination. Sight can be improved or saved by regular examinations.

Between regular eye exams, people should be aware of the symptoms of cataracts. They include:

- Faded colors
- Cloudy or blurry vision
- Poor night vision
- Double vision or multiple images
- Glare from headlights, lamps, or sunlight
- Halos around lights
- Frequent prescription changes in eyeglasses or contact lenses

Any of these symptoms should be a signal to see an eye doctor. They may be caused by cataracts or other eye disorders.

Vision depends partly on the ability of the lenses to change shape. When the lenses can no longer change shape enough to focus on near objects, presbyopia has occurred. This is common in middle age—most of those over the age of 40, and nearly all of those over 55, need glasses for reading. Reading glasses, prescription or not, may correct presbyopia.

Tearing of the eyes may arise from changes in light, temperature, or wind. Though wearing sunglasses may stop the tearing, at times a more serious condition (such as infection or a blockage of a tear duct) can cause it. In that case, professional help is called for.

The eyelids can itch, become swollen or red, or the eyelashes can become crusted during sleep. This condition (blepharitis) can be eased with warm compresses. Drugs or surgery may be needed for growths or swelling.

Floaters, the tiny specks that seem to drift across the visual field, are often a normal aspect of aging. If many new floaters appear or are accompanied by flickers of light, they can be symptoms of a visual disorder and should be brought to the attention of an ophthalmologist.

Vision exams usually include tests for high intraocular pressure, which can contribute to glaucoma, but increased intraocular pressure is only one of several factors that cause the disease. (In one type of glaucoma, intraocular pressure is normal. So a finding of normal intraocular pressure does not necessarily mean that glaucoma is not present.) Glaucoma damages the optic nerve that connects the retina to the brain, usually by increasing pressure on the nerve.

People over age 60, especially African Americans, are in a high risk group for glaucoma. Anyone who is 65 or older should be tested for glaucoma every 6 to 12 months. The ophthalmologist will test the eyes both for increased intraocular pressure and for any abnormal appearance of the retina. These tests are painless. Thickness of the cornea can affect the results of tests for glaucoma, and so the doctor should be aware of how thick the patient's cornea is. Advanced retina imaging tests are also available.

If not diagnosed and treated, glaucoma can lead to blindness. It blinds even some treated patients, but the percentage of all glaucoma patients who lose their eyesight despite treatment is only about 10%. There is no cure for glaucoma, and lost vision cannot be regained, but drugs can be given to slow its progress and alleviate the symptoms (Glaucoma Research Foundation, 2010).

CHAPTER 4

Making Informed Medical Decisions

The family doctor of the early 20th century has nearly disappeared for a variety of reasons. Today most people are cared for by medical specialists who concentrate on certain areas of the body or certain diseases.

There was a time when a doctor could carry common items—stethoscope, alcohol, aspirin, and so on—in a small black bag. In the office, it was possible to do blood and urine tests with a microscope and some simple laboratory equipment.

Today every physician has been trained to do or to order elaborate tests that were unheard of 100 years ago, to refer patients to specialists in various organs and disorders, and to prescribe a bewildering array of drugs and other treatments. Making house calls is nearly impossible, and often a general physician's office is only the first stop for patients needing care. For example, a patient who has suffered a heart attack may be referred to a cardiologist. If further treatment is needed, the cardiologist may refer the patient to a vascular surgeon. An endocrinologist becomes part of the team if the patient has diabetes as well as heart disease. Other specialists may enter the picture, also.

Specialization makes it possible to get extremely good care, but it can also lead to a fragmented approach to treatment. If there is no communication among specialists, a patient may receive medicines that nullify or conflict with each other or get advice from one specialist that interferes with advice from another. Also, specialists may not provide the preventive care that many patients need; they are more likely to enter the picture after a patient is already seriously ill.

WORKING WITH A PRIMARY PROVIDER

For elderly patients, the ideal physician might be a geriatrician who acts as the primary care provider. All care would begin with and be coordinated by the geriatrician. Because that situation is impossible for many persons, the patient or his family needs to take the initiative in coordinating care.

When seeing a doctor, especially for the first time, the patient should arrive with records of past treatments and surgeries and an up-to-date list of all medicines (including over-the-counter medicines and dietary supplements); an example is shown in Table 4.1. Names, addresses, and telephone numbers of all the patient's physicians should be given to each physician. This record will be useful if the patient needs certain laboratory tests or is treated in an emergency room.

Choosing a family doctor is one of the most crucial choices a person can make, but often the choice is a casual one based on location of the doctor's office, a recommendation by an acquaintance, or an ad in the phone book. The National Institute on Aging suggests a more organized approach. (It may be more lengthy than most people can manage but will help as an initial guide.) It advises people to begin by asking trusted friends and coworkers, health professionals, and other sources for the names of doctors they use and like. Sometimes the name of one doctor will come up several times, or people mention doctors to avoid. These conversations should lead to a tentative list of a few doctors. (Anyone who belongs to a managed care plan will

Table 4.1 A Sample Record of a Patient's Medicines

Drug	Physician	Dose	Frequency	Comments
Lisinopril	Dr. Judith Gershow	5-mg tablet	Once a day	May cause dizziness
Simvastatin	Dr. Jay Brandt	20-mg tablet	Once a day	Eat no grapefruit; take at bedtime
Aspirin	—	325-mg tablet	Occasional use as needed	
Vitamin C		2,000-mg tablet	At first sign of a cold	
Daily vitamin/ mineral supplement		1 tablet	Once a day	

be limited to the doctors who participate in that plan. The plan's membership services office can provide a list of participating doctors.)

A phone call to each of the potential doctors' offices can provide information about the doctors' education and training. Board-certified doctors have special training after medical school that enables them to specialize in geriatrics, internal medicine, or some other specialty. An office manager or nurse can explain office policies, such as whether a doctor accepts Medicare or Medicaid patients, and can say which hospitals the doctor can use. In further considering the short list of doctors, people should consider the office location (How far from home is it? Is there a parking lot? Is there a bus stop near the office? Must patients climb stairs to the office?). This can include the locations of laboratories or other medical facilities to which the doctor may send patients.

After making a tentative choice, the patient should make an initial appointment. Unless there is some urgent concern, the first visit should be for an ordinary physical examination or other routine matter. During the appointment, the doctor or a nurse will take a medical history, ask questions about previous health problems, and examine the patient. At this time, it is possible to get a first impression of the doctor, her office (including the staff), and other factors that may affect a decision. If something seems wrong, it is time for caution. It is a good idea to make an appointment for an initial appointment with another doctor. In making the initial evaluation, the patient should consider communication. (Does the doctor listen carefully, avoid using esoteric medical terms, and answer any questions? Or does he seem to ignore the patient's concerns?) If the doctor is in a group practice or relies on a nurse practitioner for examining patients, the other providers should be assessed, if possible. In some group practices, the primary doctor may be seen only occasionally.

Although privacy and confidentiality are important, in many cases a spouse or other family member can help by reminding the patient of concerns to discuss with the doctor or by taking notes while the patient is being examined. If it seems desirable to take a family member along to office visits, the doctor should be asked whether that is permissible and whether the doctor will talk to the family member about the patient's condition. The patient may or may not welcome sharing her information with family members.

Sometimes it is possible to gauge whether a doctor will be appropriate by looking at other patients in the waiting room and chatting casually with them. Are there some geriatric patients? If they volunteer any information, do they seem to have health problems that are common to the elderly?

To make the best use of limited time with a physician, a patient should have one or two definite reasons for the visit. Letting the physician know these purposes immediately helps both the physician and the patient keep the visit on track. Also, it is important to review the reasons at the end of the visit. Has the physician answered any questions about them? The patient should know what will come next—a conference with a specialist? Laboratory or X-ray studies? What are the studies for, and how will they be done? Are they painful? What are the risks and benefits? What preparation (such as fasting) is needed? When will the patient get the results? Will the physician send any new information to other providers? Has a follow-up appointment been made?

Has any new medication been prescribed? What is it for? Is a generic version of it available? How much should be taken, and at what time of day? With or without food? What side effects should be watched for? Should any food, drinks, or activities be avoided? Should any other prescriptions be stopped? If a dose is forgotten, what should be done? Does the physician have any written information about the prescription that the patient can take home?

If a diagnosis has been made, the patient should ask what the diagnosis is and receive an explanation in simple language about anything he does not understand. The physician should explain what the future is likely to hold; that is, what the prognosis is. If the condition has a genetic basis, the patient needs to know that for notifying family members. Any treatment options should be explained, with their advantages and disadvantages. A clinical trial may be available for the condition. If surgery is necessary, the physician should tell the patient why it is needed, what hospital will be used, what the procedure entails, whether anesthesia will be needed, and what will happen if surgery is postponed or avoided.

If possible, the cost of any treatment should be estimated. In some cases, insurance companies require prior notification before paying for surgery or other treatments. Some patients are annoyed by being asked for their insurance information before even seeing a doctor, but this practice is beneficial to everyone. If a physician does not accept Medicare or Medicaid patients or if there is some other problem with insurance, the patient needs to know that before having even a consultation and being billed for it. Even when insurance coverage is apparently adequate, patients need to check on it before having some kinds of tests or treatments. A call to the insurance provider can elicit information about whether a procedure is covered and about how much the insurer will pay for it.

Some patients find it helpful to keep the records of their medical appointments in a notebook. For each appointment, the reasons for it are written next to the physician's name and the date. During or after the appointment, the results and recommendations are added. Any follow-up items can be useful not just at the time, but even years later. In an age of computerized medical records, it may seem that the information is being thoroughly documented, but a simple handwritten note is often remarkably useful: one specialist fails to send results to another; a laboratory sends results for one patient to another patient having the same name; the patient changes physicians; or an elderly physician retires or dies. Any of these problems can lead to chaos and delay needed medical care.

Interpreting the results of a laboratory test for blood chemistry can be confusing. Normal values for some standard tests are shown in Table 4.2. These can be compared with a patient's results and may be useful for physician–patient discussions.

Table 4.2 Normal Values for Laboratory Tests of Blood Chemistry

Sodium	134–143 millimoles/liter
Potassium	3.5–5.2 millimoles/liter
Chloride	99–109 millimoles/liter
Total carbon dioxide (CO_2)	22–32 millimoles/liter
Glucose	77–119 milligrams/deciliter
Blood urea nitrogen	6–21 milligrams/deciliter
Creatinine	0.50–1.30 milligrams/deciliter
Albumin	3.2–4.7 grams/deciliter
Globulin	2.3–3.8 grams/deciliter
Albumin/globulin ratio	1.0–1.6
Total bilirubin	0.3–2.2 milligrams/deciliter
Alkaline phosphatase	38–126 U/liter
Calcium	8.7–10.2 milligrams/deciliter
Cholesterol	112–200 milligrams/deciliter
High-density lipoproteins (HDL)	35–85 milligrams/Deciliter
Low-density lipoproteins (LDL)	80–130milligrams/deciliter
Total/HDL cholesterol ratio	2.0–5.0

Levels associated with increased risk of coronary heart disease:

1. Total/HDL cholesterol ratio > 5.0
2. Cholesterol > 200 milligrams/deciliter
3. Cholesterol > 240 milligrams/deciliter is associated with an even greater risk of coronary heart disease.
4. HDL < 35 milligrams/Deciliter
5. LDL > 130 milligrams/deciliter

Using the Web for Medical Information

In preparing for appointments with physicians, many people now go online. The World Wide Web can be a valuable source of medical information for both physicians and patients. However, one must be cautious about which sites to visit. Some sites are advertisements, some provide too little information to be useful, and others deluge the reader with technical details. Either too much or too little information can be frightening for the layperson. In general, government sites of the National Institutes of Health, the National Library of Medicine, and others written for the public are easy to understand and reliable but may not address complex, controversial issues. To research recent developments in any medical field, it is often more useful to find articles in peer-reviewed medical journals, which can be found by searching PubMed online (www.ncbi.nlm.nih.gov/pubmed/). These articles will be very informative, but they may be too complex for the average reader or may be misinterpreted. In addition, the PubMed site is a bit difficult to navigate. Medline (http://www.nlm.nih.gov/medlineplus/) provides good, reliable information and is easier to use than PubMed.

Despite its limitations, the Web can be very useful. Educating oneself about medical matters increases general knowledge and can help patients understand their specific problems.

Working with a Doctor

Fifty or 60 years ago, patients expected to show up in a family physician's office, describe their symptoms, and follow their doctor's orders without question. For many reasons, that situation has changed considerably, and geriatric patients may find the difference disconcerting. Patients today can be more assertive about what kind of treatments to have, and they are expected to have more knowledge about the human body than patients of yesterday.

Some disorders can be treated in different ways; breast cancer, for example, may require surgery, drugs, and/or radiation. A physician may strongly recommend the type of treatment, but the patient usually has some choice. The choice should be an informed one, based on reading at the library and online. The patient should be prepared to ask the physician intelligent questions about treatment alternatives, their relative advantages, and their side effects.

In our mobile society, having the same family doctor for long periods is unusual. A patient may belong to a managed care plan that does not allow a choice of doctors, for instance. People who retire may move to a new community and need to find new medical providers. Or an elderly person may move across the country to be near a son or daughter. Whatever the reason, changing from one doctor to another can bring both new opportunities and new problems. As suggested on pages 80–81, it is important to provide the new physician with as much information as possible. Old records can be requested, and some doctors will be very helpful about sending them to new physicians. However, patients should also assume the responsibility themselves. The more information they can provide about their medical histories, the better. The new doctor needs to know about allergies, surgeries, and illnesses in the past. An electronic file is easy to print out and to read, but even handwritten personal records can be photocopied and given to a new physician.

Of course, all of this is not to say that a patient should ignore a doctor's advice. Medical training and experience give physicians the valuable ability to diagnose and treat illnesses, and, in most cases, it would be foolhardy not to use their counsel.

MEDICAL SERVICES

At some point, many families must face the decision of whether to place an elderly parent in some facility or to keep them at home. The decision may rest on the parent's medical condition and on the stress being felt by the family. Usually the parent resists leaving a familiar home, fearing that it may be the first step toward a grim nursing home. However, an assisted living facility can be very pleasant, and some people find living there preferable to remaining at home. Some residents are surprised and wish they had not resisted the move.

The choice depends partly on the elderly person's personality. A sociable man or woman can find companions for walking, playing cards, or other activities by giving up their own home and entering a group situation. That outcome is very desirable. But someone who prefers reading and writing in solitude to being with others may be willing to make many sacrifices in order to remain at home, even if the situation becomes dangerous or life-threatening. Such wishes should be respected.

Some people opt to remain at home and hire help with household chores, running errands, and other tasks that become difficult as they age. This can work well if the helpers are honest and reliable, but it may not be an option for those with little retirement money. Anyone considering hiring in-home help should be very cautious about checking references. It is easy tor a trusted helper to take advantage of an employer, especially if no other family member is on the scene.

Many people manage to spend their lives in their own homes, with about 90% of the elderly living alone entirely or with occasional help from family members or friends. At some point, however, some of the elderly find living alone too difficult. They can no longer drive, buses may not serve their neighborhoods, they develop new health problems, or some other problem arises. Often they try to continue living in their homes despite everything, but their children become concerned about the situation. Hiring a cleaning service or handyperson can help, but, eventually, the family may begin to consider the possibility of a nursing home or other living situation.

Nursing Homes and Assisted Living

The transition from a private home to assisted living can be traumatic. Few people want to give up their independence, and it may be necessary to give up valued possessions as well. However, assisted living can be quite pleasant, without the negative connotations of a nursing home. It resembles a retirement community. The resident may live in an apartment or cottage and have a kitchenette and private bathroom. In many cases, at least one meal per day is provided, leaving the resident free to prepare light meals at other times. There may be exercise and art classes. Entertainment is common; local singers and instrumentalists tend to charge less or even volunteer their talents, and there may be frequent trips to theaters and concerts. Transportation to shopping malls and other places is usually provided for residents. There is usually no regular medical care, but a nurse may be on the staff, and residents can continue seeing their regular family doctors. Unless there is some medical reason why a resident cannot leave the premises, they can go out, alone or with family members.

There is no Medicare coverage for assisted living, and so residents or their families must pay the costs themselves. Although the cost is less than that for a nursing home, it is fairly expensive and can use up a lifetime of modest savings. However, there is much variation in cost; religious organizations, for example, may provide subsidized housing for their members and religious leaders. Subsidized housing is available in some cities for those with low incomes. Anyone interested in assisted living should inquire about possible help with costs.

Some assisted living facilities are very homelike, with only a few residents sharing a large home and receiving aid with meals, bathing, and other needs. These tend to be less expensive than larger facilities, and some people prefer the family-like atmosphere. Usually fewer classes and other advantages are provided, which may be a deciding factor for or against the facility.

Some facilities provide specialized care for patients with dementia or other special needs who cannot function in other living situations. Alzheimer's patients, especially, need to be protected from wandering away from the facility. In other respects, their residences may be like any assisted living facility until they become ill enough to require skilled nursing care.

The highest level of care is a skilled nursing facility, where the atmosphere is usually much like that in a hospital. Charge nurses are registered nurses who supervise patient care and report to doctors who are associated with the facility. Certified nursing assistants or nurses' aides are well-trained assistants who are responsible for residents' daily care. They bathe the patients, help them use the toilet, push their wheelchairs, and generally help with any other needs. In skilled nursing facilities, private rooms are rare; most patients share a room and bathroom with one or two others. For many people, the lack of privacy is a significant drawback, but the need for skilled nursing may make it necessary.

Both assisted living and skilled nursing facilities may offer physical therapy, occupational therapy, speech therapy, and psychological services in varying degrees. There is usually a social services department that helps residents and families deal with insurance, government assistance such as Medicaid, and other matters. A dispensary is the source of prescriptions, which usually are brought to residents by nurses as needed. Many large homes have on-site beauty salons and exercise rooms that are helpful physically and psychologically.

Facilities of all types tend to be highly decorated, especially at holiday times, with pictures and furniture carefully chosen to impress visitors. There may be large lounges with expensive furniture and widescreen television sets. The patients' rooms may be much simpler and tend to be smaller than public rooms. However, many residents (or their families) manage to make their surroundings attractive and comfortable. Most homes encourage patients to bring family photos and to have visits from well-behaved family pets. A few nursing homes have live-in cats and caged birds that entertain patients. Patios and courtyards are often beautifully landscaped. (In choosing a home, it is helpful to note whether the outdoor areas are visible from residents' rooms, whether they are wheelchair accessible, and whether residents actually use those areas. Some homes allow residents to go outdoors only if accompanied by a family member or nursing assistant. In practice, residents seldom go outdoors.)

For anyone living in an institutional setting, food becomes important. Menus are carefully planned by dietitians, and most facilities provide nourishing (if not gourmet) meals. These may not be appealing to some residents, however. The best way to evaluate the dining services is to buy several meals at different times—preferably not on holidays, when families are visiting and meals may be much better than usual.

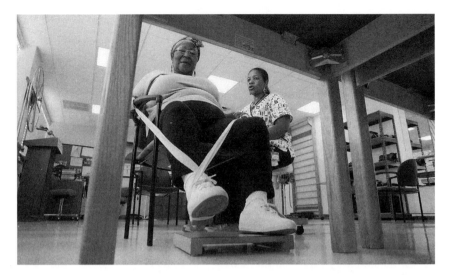

Figure 4.1   Elmaze Joseph, left, works with therapist Jocelyne Denis doing foot exercises at the Miami Jewish Home and Hospital. In addition to housing the elderly, many facilities in the United States provide rehabilitation and physical therapy to patients in their homes or in assisted living. (AP Photo/J Pat Carter.)

Choosing the right home in the beginning is very important, because making a change later may be difficult: The resident's health may deteriorate, there may be a change in her financial situation, or another home in the area may seem more appealing but cost more. Once settled, a resident may find it hard to leave an environment that is familiar, even if the environment seems undesirable. Even moving from one room to another in the same facility may be stressful.

Making the choice should not be done quickly, but too often it does happen that way. A patient is discharged from a hospital and is not ready to return home, so he is sent to a nursing home that provides physical therapy or rehabilitation. (Medicare covers up to 100 days of care, minus deductibles, if this type of setting is needed following hospitalization. Coverage lasts only while the patient's condition is improving and ends when the condition is stabilized.) That home may not be the one he would choose voluntarily, but if he does not improve enough to go home, he may spend the rest of his life there. Ideally, anyone anticipating needing an assisted living or skilled nursing facility in the future should look around at local homes while still healthy. A senior center can usually provide a list of available homes but is unlikely to give recommendations.

One way to approach the choice benefits the community as well—visitors are welcome in most facilities, and they have a chance to see the surroundings through a resident's eyes. A resident can give visitors a candid appraisal of the care. Of course, accepting a resident's comments can be an unreliable way of assessing a home; she may resent being in a nursing home or may have a biased view for some other reason. Any comments must be taken with a grain of salt. Nevertheless, a visitor can learn a great deal without being obvious about it. A visitor who is not acquainted with any of the residents in a home may be able to do volunteer work there. Some volunteers take well-behaved dogs with them to visit residents; others read to residents or do other helpful tasks. There are seldom enough nursing assistants to do everything residents need, and visitors can do much to relieve their loneliness and boredom.

Friends and acquaintances are often good resources for advice. In many communities, it is common knowledge that one facility is far superior to others or that one is particularly bad. Doctors and nurses generally know which homes are better than others.

Medicare provides a nursing home checklist that can help with the choice. It recommends looking for Medicare and Medicaid certification (which may become necessary later, even for someone who seems able to pay for care); handicapped access; strong odors (good or bad); many food choices; residents who look well cared for; and enough staff for the number of patients. Online resources from Medicare can be found at www.medicare.gov. This site includes ratings of individual nursing homes. Licensed nursing facilities are overseen by a state ombudsman who keeps track of formal complaints against facilities and any health or safety violations. Local ombudsmen act as advocates for residents and family members if there are conflicts with a facility's staff or rules. Both levels of ombudsmen can provide unbiased information about any facility being considered.

Costs can vary greatly, even in the same community. A small assisted-living facility may cost a few thousand dollars a year, while a skilled nursing facility may cost several thousand dollars a *month*. In addition to the basic charges, a home may assess additional charges for laundry, haircuts, cable television, incontinence care, and physical or speech therapy. It is important to ask about these additional charges, which can look small but quickly add up to amounts that may be burdensome.

Several sources of payment are possible. Everyone needs to be aware that Medicare does not cover the costs of assisted living or long-term skilled nursing. It provides care in a skilled nursing facility for 100 days and for limited visits from a home health care aide after a person needing special care leaves the hospital. (The aide can help with personal care.) However, Medicare does not provide long-term care.

Long-term care insurance is available. For government and military retirees, there is a fairly affordable plan. Other plans tend to be very expensive, but if someone spends many years in a nursing home, the insurance does help. Long-term care insurance does not cover assisted living at all, and in general does not pay all of the costs of a skilled nursing facility. It supplements a pension, Social Security, and other income sources. An insurance choice that some find attractive (and that is available for government employees) offers coverage for long-term care at home rather than in a skilled nursing facility. The premiums are lower, and the benefits less, than for regular long-term care insurance.

Private pay comes out of a resident's own savings and can buy very good assisted living. When those savings are exhausted, Medicaid may take over the coverage for a skilled nursing facility, but this is not guaranteed, especially in the current economic environment. Medicaid may cover some assisted living or home care costs; this varies in different states. Each state determines who qualifies for Medicaid, and even those who are approved may have to wait three months or longer. If it seems possible that Medicaid will be needed eventually, a patient or family member should check with a local office and perhaps submit an application well ahead of time.

Veterans who have serious disabilities connected to their service may qualify for skilled nursing care at U.S. Department of Veterans Affairs medical centers or at private nursing homes. The Web site (www.va.gov or 1-800-827-1000) can provide specific information about help that is available.

Whatever kind of residence is chosen, it is important for the resident to plan ahead. Facilities are likely to raise the rent and other costs periodically, just as landlords can do. In making the initial agreement with a facility (especially if a large, nonrefundable deposit is required), a potential resident should make sure that there is some restriction on how much costs can rise.

Even when costs remain the same, the quality of care in a facility can decline. New owners may acquire a facility, or the current owners may try to increase their profits by buying cheaper foods for the residents, for example. Residents cannot do much about this problem, though they or their families can lodge a complaint with the state if health or safety is affected. (For example, facilities may be legally bound to have a certain ratio of staff to patients.) If a home's quality of care continues to worsen, some residents may decide to move elsewhere if moving is feasible.

Home care by a family member or close friend may be a good solution for some people. In fact, the vast majority of the disabled elderly who are not in institutions depend on caregiving by family and friends. Because a paid arrangement affects the income taxes of both the patient and the caregiver, they should be careful to create a legal, written agreement stating how much the caregiver is paid, and payments should be made by check. If these payments sufficiently reduce the patient's assets, it may help qualify them for Medicaid and additional home care. The payments must not exceed those charged by home care agencies; even so, there are several financial advantages to this arrangement. In addition, the patient may be much happier in a home setting than in a nursing home.

However, some caution is in order: If the patient must be lifted, for instance, the caregiver must be strong enough to do so. Caregiving is a difficult job that should not be undertaken lightly or by someone with no experience. The caregiver is affected by all the issues affecting any caregiver and may feel trapped in the situation because his income now depends on it.

Whether to purchase long-term care insurance is a controversial topic: It all depends. Few nursing home residents stay in a facility for more than two or three years. Most plans are very expensive; if a person began paying the premiums in their 50s and entered a skilled nursing facility 30 years later, the premiums could far exceed the benefit. In that case, the money might better be invested. For government employees, the premiums are much more reasonable. A person with this type of policy might be able to collect as much as she paid in premiums.

The specter of having too little money for needed long-term care frightens some into buying an expensive policy. However, critics point out that, when a resident's funds are exhausted, Medicaid takes over, and there is no danger of being thrown out onto the street. Others counter that argument by saying they never want to depend on the government for support—they want to be responsible for their own care. In addition, the process of applying for Medicaid is sometimes long and difficult, and in the present troubled economy, it may become more so.

Whether someone needs care at a given level is measured partly in terms of his ability to care for himself in bathing, dressing, toileting, taking medicines, feeding, and so on. These are called activities of daily living.

A nursing home can be supportive in many ways. Residents receive medical care, physical therapy, occupational therapy, and other aids for their physical well-being. However, it can be destructive to a person's mental state, leading to infantilization of a once-intelligent man or woman. A major aspect of the infantilizing environment is the treatment of residents as children rather than as adults. In a distortion of their caregiving role, staff members may use residents' first names, speak in a sing-song tone, pitch their voices too high, and generally act in a condescending fashion.

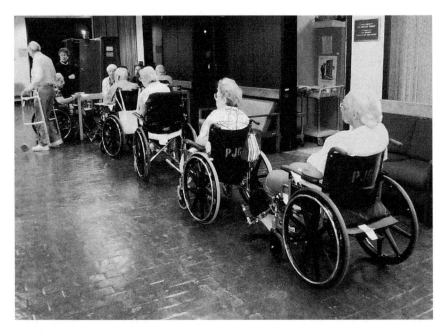

Figure 4.2 Nursing homes can be very supportive. This polling place in New Hyde Park, New York, was set up for the Parker Geriatric Institute's long-term residents, who felt that casting absentee ballots left them disconnected from the political process. (AP Photo/Kathy Willens.)

This problem is not inevitable. In her study of 50 members of a nursing home staff, doctoral student Erin Cassidy (1997) found that staff members who had been educated in the aging process, had appropriate attitudes toward older people, and were experienced in working with elderly patients were seen as more nurturing and respectful by patients than were staff members who had less education and experience. The more education the patient had, the greater their perception that staff members were disrespectful or non-nurturing.

Cassidy's study was limited to nurses and nursing assistants, but physicians are also guilty in some cases of treating their elderly patients as rather dim-witted children instead of as responsible adults. One physician treating an elderly woman was heard to say, "Doctor wants to be told that you had a good poop!" Others may ignore the patient entirely, addressing their questions to the accompanying caregiver, even though the patient is capable of hearing and understanding. Or physicians may use very abstract terms to describe a medical condition, then look annoyed or impatient if the patient asks for clarification. Cassidy's study results indicate that the training of physicians and nurses should include some obvious lessons in treating patients as adults and addressing them with respect.

End-of-Life Issues

Whether in the prime of life or at an advanced age, everyone must die. Although the prospect of death is usually unappealing, the elderly at least have the advantage of being able to do some planning. Anyone who reaches retirement age should have a life insurance policy, a will, and whatever other financial documents will be needed by their survivors or those with power of attorney.

Even with the best planning, end-of-life issues are apt to emerge unexpectedly. An acute illness may strike suddenly, or a beloved partner may die. Such events can lead one to look forward to dying.

Suicide   Some of the elderly, especially those with painful, terminal illnesses, may hope to end their lives rather than continue living as they are. Whether they follow through and commit suicide depends on their religious and other moral values; for many, suicide violates their principles and is unthinkable. Others may want to kill themselves but lack the courage or the means to do so. Still others, in numbers that are unknown but are probably large, do commit suicide rather than die in suffering.

Non-Hispanic whites commit suicide at a higher rate than other groups, with elderly men being especially vulnerable. According to the National Institute of Mental Health (2010), for every 100,000 people aged 65 or more in each of the following ethnic groups, the rate of deaths by suicide is:

- Non-Hispanic whites, 15.8
- Asian and Pacific Islanders, 10.6
- Hispanics, 7.9
- Non-Hispanic blacks, 5.0

Suicide is not always committed in solitude. The Hemlock Society was a national self-help group of people who informed themselves about methods of suicide and supported each other in making decisions about ending life. The members learned about methods that are most likely to lead to a quick death with the least pain for themselves and for their survivors (Humphry, 1991).

The Hemlock Society was formed in 1980 by Derek Humphry, who had helped his first wife to end her life. Jean Humphry was ill with cancer and had no hope of recovering. She took an overdose of drugs provided by a sympathetic doctor through Humphry. After that experience, he devoted himself to the Hemlock Society and to writing books (such as *Final Exit*) for those considering suicide. Though assisted suicide has been legal in Oregon, where he lives, since 1997, so far it is legal in only two other states—Washington and Montana—in the United States. (In other countries, it is legal only in the Netherlands and Switzerland.) He has also championed "death with dignity" legislation that would legalize euthanasia, an even more controversial subject than suicide.

As might be expected, those in the right-to-life anti-abortion movement strongly opposed the Hemlock Society, because they thought it encouraged suicide. In 2004, the Hemlock Society disbanded and joined with Aid in Dying and similar groups to form the Compassion and Choices support group. Members support each other, educate people about choices, and advocate for improved laws. Its Web site emphasizes the groups' opposition to suicide; rather, it aids and supports the already dying who want to hasten death in order to be released from pain.

The issue is still extremely controversial, and it emerged as part of the dispute over health insurance reform in 2009, when critics of the proposed plan said that part of it amounted to "pulling the plug on Grandma."

Society has become more compassionate about suicide as more and more people have killed themselves to escape great pain for themselves and their families. When suicide is assisted by doctors and nurses, however, there is less tolerance. Physician Jack Kevorkian became notorious for assisting several patients to die. In 1999, Kevorkian was sent to prison for up to 25 years, convicted of murder after he allowed a video of an assisted suicide to be shown on national television. In 2007, he was released on parole. Kevorkian is still a controversial figure, known to some as Dr. Death and to others as a sympathetic and courageous hero.

Hospice Care   If someone is expected to have only months to live, hospice care is available. Medicare covers hospice care if the patient has a terminal illness and a doctor has certified that he or she is expected to die within six months. (Some communities have hospice centers that are free for patients of any age.) The very humane goal of hospice care is to make the dying person as comfortable and pain-free as possible. A do-not-resuscitate order, from the patient or someone having medical power of attorney, prevents the use of any measures that would prolong life. Only palliative care is allowed. This includes drugs for pain relief and symptom management; medical, nursing, and social services; and some services that are not covered by Medicare, such as grief counseling.

In some cases, the person receives hospice care at home. A visiting nurse comes in often to give any needed injections and to supervise conditions.

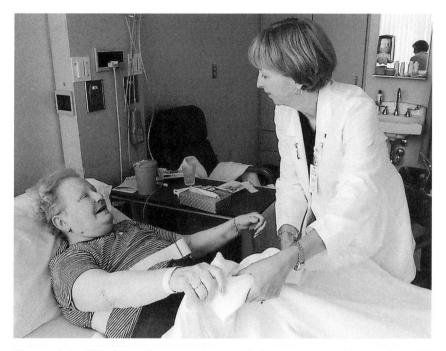

Figure 4.3   Hospice patients are given palliative care to provide comfort. (AP Photo/Michael Reigner.)

The patient is in familiar surroundings with family members near by, and some respite care is provided to give the caregivers relief from continuing responsibility.

Some hospice patients spend their last days in a nursing home or special hospice center. Like those receiving home care, they are given palliative care only. Medicare covers inpatient respite care, care given in a Medicare-approved facility to give the usual caregiver a chance to rest. (Each time the patient receives respite care, she can stay in the facility for five days.) Medicare also will pay for covered services for health problems that are unrelated to the terminal illness. Hospice care can continue as long as a hospice medical director or doctor recertifies that the patient is terminally ill. No matter where hospice care is given, it provides a chance for the patient to make a will or other legal arrangements, to make amends, to express any wishes about a funeral or final resting place, and to do anything else that seems necessary.

CHAPTER 5

Social and Psychological Issues

LIVING ARRANGEMENTS FOR THE ELDERLY

The elderly need community support, both in terms of where they live and in terms of who shares their lives. Close relatives, spouses, or friends may become caregivers.

Caregiving

Caregiving can be satisfying for caregivers, despite its demands on their time and energy. In some cases, marriages are made stronger or parent–child bonds are restored when a family member is ill or dying. A person who has led a fairly selfish life may respond to being a caregiver by behaving altruistically. Like parenting, caregiving can lead to new knowledge and skills.

On the other hand, caregiving that continues for a long period can be extremely stressful. The caregiver may become physically ill or fatigued and may be impatient and angry. Caregivers may come to resent the people they love—both the patient and other family members. Preventing those results is important for everyone concerned.

The slide into long-term caregiving is often gradual. One person (often a daughter) becomes more and more responsible for another, and other family members may not offer any help. At the first sign that that is happening, the caregiver needs to assert her need for respite and aid. Otherwise, the situation is likely to become much worse.

Frequent breaks can help—even a short walk with the family dog can get the caregiver out of the house and lead to needed contact with neighbors. Trips to stores and libraries are necessary reasons to get away, also.

If the patient can be left alone for brief periods, these breaks are easily arranged; if not, a neighbor or paid helper may be recruited to stay while the caregiver goes out. (Often people will offer to shop for a caregiver out of a misguided desire to help, not realizing that running errands can be beneficial.)

Once a week or so, any caregiver needs a longer break—an afternoon matinee, a long shopping trip, an evening out with friends, or some other time away from continual caregiving. This time can be as restorative as a short vacation.

Many caregivers become isolated as time goes on, spending most of the time with the patient. Less and less time is spent with friends, at religious services, and at community events. To avoid isolation, caregivers need to remain part of social groups, and possibly to continue working part-time outside the home. (This can help the family financially as well, and the money is often needed.) Some religious congregations offer aid, and there are many caregivers' support groups. Caregivers have a continuing need to express their concerns to friendly, supportive listeners.

When a patient cannot leave home, that can become an opportunity to invite friends to visit. It is not necessary to give dinner parties, which might add to the caregiver's burdens; a simple evening of games, conversation, or working on hobbies can be stimulating for the patient and enjoyable for everyone. (For instance, during the final years of one magician's life, some of his fellow magicians spent occasional evenings with him, practicing their tricks on each other and telling jokes. It meant a great deal to him and to his caregiver wife.)

In caring for the patient, some caregivers neglect their own health. To avoid this, they need to plan healthy meals, exercise, get enough sleep, and visit medical providers as needed. Following these suggestions may be difficult, but it is not selfish. If the caregiver becomes burned out, his ability to care for the patient is diminished. In addition, the caregiver may become angry with the patient and with other family members.

If the patient is left alone at times, the caregiver should leave emergency information where a neighbor, household worker, or other person will see it. The following is an example of useful information that might be left:

Emergency Information for John Doe

John has type 1 diabetes. If his blood sugar drops too far, he will seem drunk and disoriented. He usually needs only to eat about a teaspoonful of sugar or to drink half a cup of orange juice. If he doesn't recover after 10 minutes, give him the same amount of sugar or orange juice and wait 10 minutes more. If that doesn't help, call 911.

Information for EMT or Hospital:
Medicines
    Prescriptions:

Simvastatin	20 mg/day
Lisinopril	20 mg/day

    Insulin:

Regular (Novolin R)	15 to 19 units 2 or 3 times per day
Levimir (overnight)	33 units every night
Fast-acting (Novolog)	10 to 19 units if needed for high blood sugar

    Over-the-counter:
    Multivitamin/mineral comb. (Centrum Silver type) one per day

Aspirin	81 mg/day

Phone numbers:
    Jane Doe xxx–xxxx, or cell xxx–xxxx
    Jim Smith (neighbor) xxx–xxxx
    Debbie Jones (sister) xxx–xxxx

The primary caregiver's burden can be reduced greatly by willing friends. Unfortunately, too often those considering a visit to a nursing home or other home of the elderly sick react with, "Those places depress me too much—I can't go there." They might do well to consider how depressing "those places" can be for the residents and for caregivers who spend many hours there. An occasional visit, or even a mailed greeting card, can help enormously and takes little effort.

Those who visit nursing homes daily learn to make the most of their visits. They advise visitors to use strategies like these:

- Visit at a good time of day for the resident, such as mid-morning or mid-afternoon, rather than at mealtime. Ask the resident or primary caregiver about the best time to visit.
- Plan your visit ahead of time. Learn the resident's schedule for exercise, art classes, or other enjoyable activities to avoid interrupting them.
- Find out about any dietary restrictions, and obey them. The charge nurse can suggest treats that are allowed for the resident.
- Take the resident outdoors if possible. Even in winter, you may find a sheltered, sunny spot. Many residences have lovely gardens or patios that are used for impressing visitors but are seldom enjoyed by residents.

- Be prepared to entertain yourself with a book or magazine if the resident is sleeping or otherwise unavailable for a while.
- Make your visits short. More than an hour may be tiring for the resident and difficult emotionally for you.
- Encourage the resident to attend any musical or other event taking place during your visit. You also will be welcome there, and may find it unexpectedly enjoyable.
- Make any gifts small and useful. Most residences have extremely small rooms, with no space for tchotchkes. Some gifts that are welcomed by many are large-print books, recent magazines, and (if permitted) fresh fruit, candy, or ice cream. If you take flowers, provide a vase, or take a well-watered plant. Do not expect anyone to care for flowers after you leave.
- Find out whether the resident needs toiletries such as deodorant and toothpaste. Although these are commonly provided by nursing homes, they may be very cheap brands that the resident dislikes. A bar of soap, bottle of hand lotion, or box of tissues in the resident's favorite brand can be a welcome gift.
- Think of your visit as a pleasant time, not a chore. Think ahead about how you can make it enjoyable. For instance, perhaps you have a photo album or a laptop computer with images that you and the resident can look at together. She may enjoy hearing the latest gossip about mutual acquaintances.
- Do not be an unwelcome visitor. The resident probably has a roommate who may want to sleep or to have a quiet room. Be especially careful not to take a large, noisy group to visit at the same time. This can be tiring for the resident, irritating to a roommate, and a problem for the nurses.
- Leaving can be the most difficult part of a visit, especially if the resident becomes tearful or begs you to return soon. To make leaving easier, make an appointment ahead of time, so that you can honestly say you must leave at a certain hour. Mention the appointment when you arrive. When you leave, do not promise to visit again unless you actually will do so.

If the elderly person must have surgery or enter a hospital for some reason, the caregiver's role changes. In some ways, it becomes easier: Rather than bearing the complete burden of responsibility for the patient, the caregiver is helped by doctors, nurses, technicians, and other hospital workers. Suddenly it is possible to leave the patient for several hours or overnight. This can remove much stress from the caregiver's daily life.

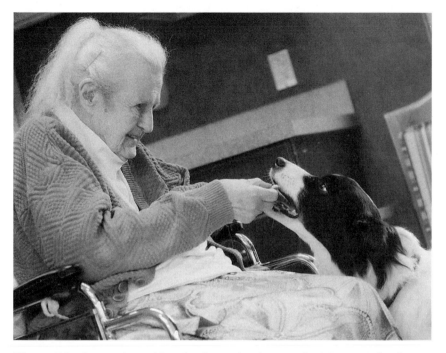

Figure 5.1 Interacting with animals can be therapeutic. Many nursing homes encourage visits by well-behaved animals and may have resident pets as well. (AP Photo/Mike Groll.)

On the other hand, new responsibilities are added. Depending on the seriousness of the patient's condition, the caregiver may need to stay in the hospital room much of the time. Even in the best facilities, mistakes can be made, and so the caregiver needs to be vigilant about the foods, medicines, and therapies the patient is receiving. Visitors or the patient's roommate may be noisy or otherwise interfere with the patient's recovery. If the patient is deaf, doctors and nurses may not bother to write notes of explanation, which can frighten the patient; the caregiver can help by asking questions, listening carefully, and giving the patient any needed information. Sometimes medical personnel can be told to speak into a patient's right ear or otherwise make the patient hear them, but this may help only at the moment. If the patient is not a native English speaker, the caregiver may need to translate.

Because of the Health Insurance Portability and Accountability Act (HIPAA) of 1996, hospitals guard patients' privacy to a degree that sometimes becomes frustrating for families and friends. Though HIPAA was passed for good reasons, charge nurses will not provide information to just anyone who calls to ask about a patient's condition. This means that the caregiver is likely to receive calls instead. To preserve their own sanity, many caregivers have learned to establish boundaries. Instead of interrupting their work and answering the telephone immediately, they let calls go to voice mail or answering machines. (In addition, they can post updates on the patient's condition on these machines, which is convenient both for the caregivers and for anxious callers.)

Hospital-acquired infections such as those caused by methicillin-resistant *Staphylococcus aureus* are common, and the elderly sick are especially vulnerable to them. Unfortunately, many medical personnel—to say nothing of casual visitors—fail to wash or sanitize their hands as they enter or leave hospital rooms. Any bacteria on their hands may reach patients. The caregiver can protect the patient by diplomatically reminding people to prevent spreading infections by washing their hands.

At the time of discharge, the caregiver should be present to get all needed instructions (both oral and written) for the patient's follow-up appointments and home care. Even if fully recovered, the patient may be distracted by whatever is going on during the discharge, which interferes with processing that important information.

Cooperative Aging

Elderly widows have been common in all societies throughout history, and that has not changed. Today, though, many widows and widowers are healthy and energetic and are unwilling to remain alone or to move in with their children. If they reach the stage of acceptance after losing their spouses and can find compatible new partners, they are likely to remarry. Those whose marriages ended in divorce may be optimistic enough to marry again.

Remarriage can be a happy event for the new couple but may lead to problems as well. If each partner had previously had a long marriage or relationship, during which there were many years of adjusting to each other and sharing experiences, it can be difficult to live with a new person—however compatible—whose previous life was quite different. Toward the end of life, there are too few years available for adaptation and for sharing new experiences. As one elderly widow wisecracked, "I'm not going to marry again—it takes about seven years just to break in a husband!"

In early marriages, people cooperate to reach goals of raising children, building a home together, and so on. Later, those goals have been reached (Zoler, 2008). New challenges confront elderly couples, whether they have been married for many years or are newly remarried.

When the elderly of today were young, it was common for a wife not to work outside the home or to do so only long enough to put her husband through school, and that became the focus of the couple's first few years of marriage. The next stage was usually devoted to having babies and raising a family. In middle age, many women returned to school themselves, and that became another major objective.

Older couples have different goals, which may or may not be shared. A husband and wife may both enroll in lifelong learning classes, which are enjoyable but not focused on career goals. They may have time at last for their special leisure pursuits, such as painting, studying philosophy, fishing, learning a foreign language, or collecting model railroad trains. Unlike younger couples, whose goals are largely imposed by societal conventions, an older couple can freely explore their individual interests.

Both partners in an elderly marriage are likely to have medical issues, or at least to be working on improving their health and fitness. It is important for them to support each other in visiting doctors, keeping records, exercising, and picking up prescriptions and using them correctly. They may need different diets than when they were younger, and they may have established definite food preferences. Cooperation in an elderly marriage

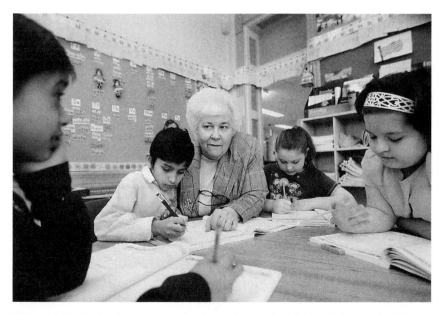

Figure 5.2   Retired teachers and other retirees often find satisfaction in helping young learners. (AP Photo/Cheryl Senter.)

is not limited to medical and health issues. They need each other for many reasons of companionship, emotional support, sex, and security.

Some men find retirement difficult at first but adjust to the situation over time. In a seven-year study of 117 retired Canadian men, Gall et al. (1997) found that most of the men responded positively to retirement during the first year, and their psychological health and general well-being increased even more over the succeeding years. In the short term, physical health and sufficient income led to a positive adjustment, as did voluntarily retiring (rather than involuntarily retiring). Those who perceived their situation as under their control also found it easier to adjust to retirement, both in the first year and after seven years.

A man's retiring can make life difficult for his partner. A man who has traveled frequently in his work or who has been absent from home part of every day, suddenly is there most of the time. He may follow his wife when she goes shopping, or he may want to have lunch with her when she might

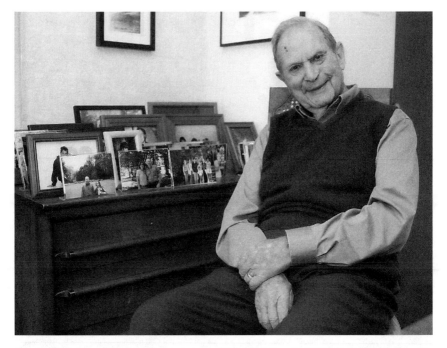

Figure 5.3 Ken Wilde, 86, received an MA in history in 2009 from the University of Missouri–St. Louis. Lifelong learning gives many older people energy and purpose. (AP Photo/Tom Gannam.)

prefer to meet some women friends for lunch and spend the afternoon at a museum or a movie. She must choose between hurting his feelings and losing an important part of her own social life. Letters to advice columnists are often written by women who find themselves in this predicament.

Even if a man's retirement is satisfying, unmarried elderly men are likely to be unhealthy. According to the Israeli Ischemic Heart Study (a study of more than 10,000 Israeli men beginning in 1963 and ending in 1997), a single elderly man is 64% more likely than a married man to have a fatal stroke. In addition, satisfaction in marriage makes a great difference: Unhappily married men are also 64% more prone to strokes than happily married men (Goldbourt et al., 2010).

Elderly men adjust to being single with much more difficulty than elderly women do. (Women may speculate with some amusement on the explanation for the difference, but current research leaves the reasons unclear.) Some elderly single men begin behaving bizarrely or become suicidal. According to the National Institutes of Health, the elderly have the highest rate of suicide in any age group. Men, especially older men, are more likely than women to choose violent methods of suicide, such as shooting themselves. For that reason, their suicide attempts are more likely to be accomplished.

Elderly women may fare better than men when it comes to dealing with health and loneliness, but they have a greater problem with poverty. Many elderly women worked only a few years, or worked at low-paying jobs, so they paid little into Social Security. Because Social Security income is based on the best years of earnings, such women have lower benefits than men or women who paid more into the system.

Even those who collect the maximum Social Security benefits may struggle to make ends meet. A widow who was a caregiver for her husband through years of an expensive illness may have stopped working during those years and used her own retirement savings to take care of him. They may have had to sell their home. Unless her husband left plenty of life insurance or otherwise provided for her, as a widow, she is likely to be living on Social Security alone. To pay her bills, she may have to share a home or apartment with someone else.

Elderly women are more apt to live independently if they are able financially to do so. A study by Engelhardt et al. (2005) showed that when Social Security benefits rose in the 1980s, elderly widows depending on Social Security were more likely to live alone; when a cutback in benefits occurred in the 1990s, they were more likely to adopt shared living arrangements. The impact on divorcées, the fastest-growing part of the elderly population, was even greater. In conclusion, the authors stated that if Social Security benefits were cut by 10%, more than 600,000 independent elderly households would move into shared living arrangements.

Some elderly pairs choose to marry, but others stay single and share living quarters with partners. That arrangement seemed shocking at one time but is now accepted in all but the most conservative parts of the country. The baby boomers' casual lifestyles included living together without marriage, and many of the aging boomers continue that custom.

In part, cohabiting is the result of dependence on Social Security and Medicaid; some of those who stay single would lose needed financial and medical benefits if they married. Rather than becoming impoverished, they forgo marriage, even if they desire it.

Sometimes the children of elderly people raise objections for financial considerations to their parents remarrying. For instance, the children may fear that they will lose an expected inheritance. A prenuptial agreement is a wise precaution for couples with children as well as for couples whose incomes or assets are unequal.

Some couples find it difficult to decide where to live if they remarry or cohabit. If each partner already has a home and wants to remain in it, some compromises are necessary. In some cases, they retain both homes and live in one for part of the year and the other during the other part. This may work out well, or it may lead to arguments about which home is better or located in a more desirable area.

Many elderly people want to go on living in a single-family house, even if it is too large for them and difficult to clean and maintain. Others may choose to move into a rented apartment or a condominium. Still others may hit the road, buying a recreational vehicle and traveling. The choice depends on their personal preferences for a lifestyle and on what they can afford.

Cohousing is an attractive choice for some retirees. A housing model that began in Denmark in the 1960s, these small communities are planned, designed, built, managed, maintained, and loved by people of all ages who live in them. This option is more widespread in western Europe, where there are between 700 and 1,200 such communities, mainly in Denmark; because of its many advantages, it may become more popular in the United States. At this time, there are at least 110 cohousing communities in the United States, only 3 of which are for seniors only. However, the elderly are welcome residents in every group. A variety of families and single people live in apartments, condominiums, townhouses, or small homes. They also jointly own common facilities where they share several meals each week, and perhaps a laundry, workshop, guest rooms, meeting spaces, and (where there are children) a play room. These communities are self-governed, and the management and maintenance work are shared by the residents. This alternative is not economical, because the homes sell for prevailing rates in the area. However, residents find them a neighborly, supportive environment that is an excellent value for the price.

Cohousing is not a form of assisted living. Residents live independently except for the shared meals and common activities. Also, if residents lose the ability to live independently, they must move elsewhere. The Web site www.cohousing.org provides information about cohousing.

For many of the elderly, finding a partner for sharing living quarters, or even for occasional platonic companionship, is difficult. They may spend years following the usual suggestions—going to church or temple services, joining the local Friends of the Library, and getting involved in various social groups—without ever meeting anyone of interest.

Those who do find partners successfully tend to look for them at alumni reunions and in other groups where the members share some common background. (For instance, some very successful remarriages among elderly couples are between people who met originally in high school and then married different people.) Trying to find common ground with someone who grew up in a different part of the country, has different religious beliefs, or has a different educational level is difficult.

Some of the elderly are joining their young, single counterparts in online dating. While fraught with potential problems and even dangers, online dating can be an entertaining way of meeting potential friends and partners one would never meet otherwise. Though some sites focus entirely on marriage and partnerships, others emphasize meeting through common interests that can be a good basis for friendships. For instance, one online singles group invites new members by advertising on its home page that they can meet progressive singles who are environmentalists, vegetarians, or animal-rights activists and who share a global consciousness and inquisitive spirit. Another group's Web site stresses that the members are alumni of Ivy League and certain other private colleges and universities. Most sites declare that their members are a diverse group sharing common values and interests; and all mention friendship, dating, and romance. Some welcome both homosexuals and heterosexuals; others are limited to one orientation or the other.

DEATH AND MOURNING

One of the most painful parts of aging is the loss of family and friends. At each loss, the survivors must go through another grieving process.

Grief

Grieving follows different patterns in different people, but Kübler-Ross and Kessler (2005) identified five main stages that are generally traversed:

Denial. Some survivors fail to accept that the death has taken place. This usually lasts for a very short time, during which the survivor may think the dead person will come back, that there has been some mistake. Many widows and widowers find themselves talking to their dead spouses and having seemingly paranormal experiences.

Anger. "How can you die and leave me here alone?" is a common reaction to the death of a loved one. The survivor feels great anger at the dead person, at someone who seems responsible for the death, or at the entire world or at God. Some self-recrimination may be part of this phase.

Bargaining. A grief-stricken person may think it is possible to change the situation by making some bargain with God. "If I stop drinking [or behave better in some other way], can they come back?"

Depression. This stage often follows the initial weeks after a funeral. When there is no longer a lot of work to do and arrangements to be made, a survivor may feel numb. The earlier sadness and anger may still be obvious, or it may be hidden. Depression may manifest itself as anxiety or insomnia.

Acceptance. Eventually the survivor accepts the loss, even though feelings of sadness may remain permanently.

Although most survivors go through these stages, they may not occur in this order, and there are individual variations in how the stages are manifested. Some of them are irrational, but that is scarcely surprising—losing a loved one causes many survivors to behave in unreasonable and even frightening ways.

The death of a partner can have a devastating impact on an elderly person. It commonly takes at least two or three years for a widow or widower to regain equilibrium; in the meantime, they may forget the things they set out to do just a few minutes earlier, have trouble balancing checkbooks, and have difficulties in general. Their feelings of identity and self-esteem are damaged, also. It is a confusing, bewildering time during which they may wonder if they are losing their mind. Just knowing the likelihood that these events can occur can be comforting.

Friends who are sympathetic and supportive in the weeks following a death may become less so as time goes on. Single people are less likely than couples to be invited to social occasions, simply because it is less convenient for the hosts. Also, acting cheerful can be difficult for the bereaved, and no one wants to spend much time around someone who is even mildly sad much of the time.

Many widows and widowers find that close friends who have also lost their mates can be more understanding than anyone else; no one can completely understand grief before experiencing it. A close group of widowed friends can be literally lifesaving for a few years after a death.

However, in the long run, the friends may actually impede a person's recovery from a partner's death. In a study of 101 elderly persons who had lost their mates during the previous two and a half years, a Dutch researcher found that the presence of close friends increased their loneliness (van Baarsen, 2002). This effect was especially apparent in those who had low self-esteem. It may be that bereaved people become too dependent on close friends or family members, leaning on them for emotional support rather than making an effort to meet other people and proceed with their lives.

Many support groups are available to help survivors work through grief along with others who are experiencing the same kinds of loss. These groups can be more helpful than friends, because the groups may be led by experienced counselors who are not personally involved in the survivors' lives.

Funerals

Funerals become a major concern as we age, both in planning for our own deaths and in carrying out the wishes of loved ones. Some preplanning and thought about this issue can ease the pain and help to control financial costs.

What is necessary or appropriate differs considerably in various religions and communities. A minister, priest, rabbi, or imam can provide specific information about guidelines for their religious group. For those with no religious affiliation or for those who are planning a funeral or memorial service in another area, a funeral director can be a great help in finding such information and in finding someone to officiate at the service.

Whether to have a traditional funeral, complete with a wake or viewing, is sometimes problematical. In recent years, memorial services have become more common. The dead person may have already been buried or cremated before the service and is present at the service as ashes (cremains) or not at all. Those who attend may mourn openly or may eulogize the departed, trying to emphasize the person's contributions to society or to themselves personally.

A simple but dignified, moving service can cost as little as a few thousand dollars. If the body is cremated, the ashes can be placed in a wooden box that is suitable for use in the service. If the person is to be buried, there is no need for an elaborate, expensive coffin unless the family wishes it, or if the person preplanned the service and specified a certain type of coffin. Similarly, embalming is an option that may be unnecessary. (However, some cemeteries are very restrictive about how bodies or ashes are enclosed, requiring expensive containers for burial.)

Many people buy cemetery lots well before their deaths, especially if they want to be buried in a family plot. The deed to a cemetery lot should be kept in a safe deposit box or other place where survivors will find it quickly when the need arises. Additionally, a gravestone may already have been purchased.

Other details can be preplanned as well. In this technological age, some people leave videos of themselves in which they say their postmortem good-byes to friends and relatives. More commonly, people will leave instructions for the type of service they want, along with their wills and other emergency information. Perhaps even more useful are the instructions some people leave regarding the things they do *not* want at their funerals or on their graves—music they abhorred when alive, eulogies, elaborate carvings on tombstones, or anything else of personal importance. Any such final choices should be respected.

The Federal Trade Commission (FTC) has established the Funeral Rule, which governs the U.S. funeral industry and attempts to prevent expensive, unethical practices. The FTC's Web site (www.ftc.gov) contains links to other Web sites that may be needed after a death.

Planning or experiencing a funeral is always difficult emotionally, but the financial cost can be contained, and the survivors can feel they have honored the last wishes of the person who has died. There is some satisfaction in this, which helps to mitigate the pain of losing a friend or relative.

ETHICAL ISSUES

The elderly are often easy targets for those who want to take advantage of them or abuse them. Physically more frail than younger people, with failing vision or hearing, they may be unable to understand what is happening or to take defensive action. In addition, they may be socially isolated and lack a network of friends and relatives who could help them.

Fraud

People of all ages may be targets for fraud, and the Internet makes it especially easy. How many of us have not received messages from someone in Nigeria who needs to get a little help in moving some money out of the country and only needs access to our bank account information to do so? Or who has a guaranteed method of earning a lot of money for very little work? Or who wants to send us millions of dollars in lottery winnings but has to charge a small fee for doing so? Such messages arrive in endless variations, year after year. Most of us simply delete them or move them to a trash folder, but some people do fall for the scams. Because it is embarrassing to be duped, the number of people who are victimized may never be known.

A useful Web site for checking possible frauds and rumors is www. snopes.com, run by Barbara and David P. Mikkelson. The Mikkelsons check on urban legends and verify or disprove them. The site is sometimes highly entertaining as well as educational.

In the aftermath of hurricane Katrina and other disasters, unscrupulous contractors and their workers were able to prey on elderly homeowners who desperately needed help in relocating or in repairing their damaged homes. They could charge high rates for shoddy work, collect their pay, then disappear before a job was finished. Even in normal circumstances, and with younger victims, this type of abuse can occur; after a disaster, and with elderly people, it is all too common.

Financial abuse can also take the form of obvious scams like the pigeon drop, where the victim gives someone a large sum of money in the hope of getting a portion of some "found money." The victim loses their money, and the perpetrator disappears. Although the victim is partly to blame for being greedy, an impoverished elderly person may find a scam like this one very tempting.

Health-related frauds are common. For example, an elderly couple who can no longer work may be persuaded to sell an expensive nutritional product from their home. They may invest a large amount of money in the product, fill their garage with the product, and then find they are not able to sell it. Or an elderly person may pay far too much for an over-the-counter medicine that is useless or even harmful.

Abuse

Physical or emotional abuse of the elderly may come about when a hired caregiver or even a family member is cruel to a patient. The elderly person is not strong enough to stop the abuse and may be too dependent on the abuser to dare to complain to anyone who might step in to help.

More often, people are thoughtless rather than deliberately unkind in their treatment of the elderly: Physicians and other medical personnel may shout at patients with the assumption that they cannot hear; people may not be willing to wait an extra moment for an elderly person; and so on.

Physicians and others need to be alert to symptoms of abuse when working with the elderly. For instance, they may note some bruises or a fearful demeanor. Some gentle questioning may uncover a situation that should be reported to a social worker or the police. Unless a potential abuser absolutely must be present, the questioning should take place in private, so that the elderly person feels safe in divulging any damaging information. Most large cities have agencies that protect the elderly if they are notified about problems of abuse or neglect, but someone needs to bring the problems to their attention.

Neglect, without actual abuse, is probably more common. A busy caregiver, even with good intentions, may find it hard to give an elderly patient enough help with shopping, grooming, and other matters. Again, a physician may note from a patient's appearance that he or she is being neglected. It may be helpful to suggest a move to assisted living or a to make a telephone call to a local Meals on Wheels group. Many aids are available, but they must be requested. Senior centers are usually excellent sources for these referrals.

A less abusive, but very irritating, problem is the patronizing attitude of many toward the elderly. Any gray-haired woman is apt to be addressed condescendingly as "Dear," "Young lady," or "Sweetheart," for instance. Or, an only slightly younger woman will loudly insist on helping her with a grocery cart or heavy door, even though she can manage very well herself, thank you. In physicians' offices, even the very old and highly educated are addressed by their first names, but are expected to address the physician as "Doctor." The problem is somewhat similar to that encountered by feminists in the 1970s who were treated with too little courtesy or too much chivalry and who were accused of being humorless when they objected to jokes about liberated women. If an elderly person protests about unkind treatment, they may seem cranky or paranoid; rather than having that happen, they tend to say nothing.

Occasional horror stories appear in the media about elder abuse: A nursing home resident is raped, an old man is abandoned by his family in a bus station, an old woman is beaten and robbed as she walks to a grocery store. Though such tragedies do occur, fortunately they are rare. Most nursing homes are safe places where the residents' physical needs are met by a caring staff. Most families make some effort to care for their elderly members. And, in most areas, old people can leave their homes without fear of being attacked.

Nevertheless, elder abuse of varying degrees does occur. Perhaps the most common type is legal and financial abuse, because it is most likely to benefit the abuser and can be concealed more easily than physical or emotional abuse. Even those who appear safe may be victims, as shown by the shameful treatment of wealthy philanthropist Brooke Astor by her son, who siphoned off millions of dollars of her money and neglected her (Barron, 2009).

Those who want to protect the elderly from legal or financial abuse may include their lawyers, family members, friends, the clergy, bank tellers, health aides, accountants, and others who may notice something amiss in the person's bank accounts and other records. (Unfortunately, an abuser may be among this group.) The danger signs include:

- Large withdrawals from bank accounts or investments
- Sudden secrecy about legal or financial matters
- A large discrepancy between lifestyle and known assets
- A surprising change in a will

Questioning the possible victim must be done tactfully, because most people tend to be secretive about their financial status. If possible, the questioning is best done by a trusted close friend. Whoever suspects abuse can confer with others who may have more information or are likely to have their own suspicions. If there is definite evidence of abuse, it should be reported to the person or agency that can take action. Often the best person to stop the abuse is a close family member, but he or she may be unaware of the problem until someone outside the family points it out.

Physical abuse is the most obvious kind of abuse, because it often leaves visible signs. Doctors and other health professionals should note any of the following signs of possible physical abuse:

- Bruises or welts having no apparent cause
- Vaginal or anal bleeding
- Broken bones
- Wounds or cuts
- Signs of physical restraint
- Suspicious behavior by a caregiver
- A fearful attitude toward some other person

Sexual abuse can range from rape and other major physical harm to emotional abuse such as forcing an elderly person to look at pornography. Much sexual abuse may go unreported, partly because many elderly people grew up in a time when sex was a shameful subject, and they hesitate to discuss the abuse with anyone. Questioning them to elicit information must be extremely diplomatic.

Evidence of physical or sexual abuse—especially a photo—is important support for any accusations and should be taken to the police or other authorities. The Eldercare Locator, at 1-800-677-1116, can provide telephone numbers to be used in each state. If someone is in immediate danger, 911 or a local police number should be called.

CHAPTER 6

Legal and Political Issues

During the Great Depression, many elderly people lost their entire life savings. To prevent that happening again, Social Security was established in 1935, ensuring that all citizens would receive at least a small income after reaching the age of 65 or becoming disabled. Medicare was enacted in 1965, following years of opposition by the American Medical Association—which viewed it as a step toward socialized medicine—to help the elderly to pay their medical bills.

THE ELDERLY IN THE MEDICAL SYSTEM

The Social Security program is funded by deductions from the first 6.2% of a worker's gross income (up to an income of $106,800 for 2010). The employer pays an additional 6.2% that does not come out of the worker's paycheck. These funds are then invested, with the proceeds being used to pay benefits. Similarly, 1.45% of gross income is withheld from a worker's paycheck (with no income limit) to fund Medicare, and the employer pays another 1.45%. The Medicaid program (called Medi-Cal in California) provides medical and dental care for people of all ages who have few assets, such as nursing home residents who have exhausted their savings. All together, the three programs account for 40% of the federal budget (Kaiser Family Foundation, 2009).

The importance of Medicare for the elderly population was demonstrated by a longitudinal study (McWilliams et al., 2007) of thousands of elderly people on Medicare, about half of whom had been uninsured until the age of 65. Compared with people on Medicare who had been previously insured, the newly insured group reported significant improvements in agility, mobility, cardiovascular health, and general health. The improvement was especially noted for those who had diabetes or cardiovascular disease.

Medicare beneficiaries can choose between the traditional fee-for-service (FFS) program—sometimes called Original Medicare—and private health plans that include health maintenance organizations (HMOs) and preferred provider organizations (PPOs). HMOs and PPOs are part of the Medicare Advantage program.

Under FFS Medicare, beneficiaries can choose to be treated by any hospital or doctor. Medicare Advantage plans require patients to receive treatment from providers in a network or to pay a higher fee to receive care from another provider. Most Medicare Advantage plans provide all benefits covered under traditional Medicare. Today, although most Medicare beneficiaries are covered under FFS Medicare, the number enrolled in private Medicare Advantage plans has risen to nearly a quarter of Medicare's 45 million beneficiaries. In recent years, Congress has authorized generous payments to Medical Advantage plans that have resulted in this rapid growth. This payment system increases Medicare costs, reduces the solvency of the Part A trust fund, and increases Part B premiums paid by all beneficiaries (Kaiser Family Foundation, 2009). In addition to those disadvantages, some Medicare Advantage enrollees have had difficulty in collecting their benefits if they move to another state. Under the provisions of the 2010 health plan, Medicare Advantage providers may be reimbursed less in the future.

Social Security and Medicare have worked well until recent years, because the number of workers far exceeded the number of retirees, and salaries grew much larger than when the programs began. However, as the proportion of workers to retired people has lessened and the U.S. economy has suffered, it seems less certain that people can count on a secure retirement.

Can Social Security and Medicare last long enough to support the baby boomers and younger people? It appears that Social Security is safe until 2037, but benefits will have to be reduced after that if current conditions continue (Social Security and Medicare Boards of Trustees, 2010). Medicare is another matter. The cost of medical care has skyrocketed since the 1960s, and Medicare deductions and reimbursements have not risen accordingly. Only Medicare Part A is provided without cost to most of those over 65; Parts B and D are options that cost extra. Even if they purchase the options, many Medicare recipients also need to purchase Medigap insurance policies from private insurers to cover part of their medical costs. Private insurers can and do raise their rates or refuse to pay bills for enrollees who failed to disclose preexisting conditions when they enrolled. (Under the provisions of the 2010 health care reform, insurers will no longer be able to refuse payment for that reason.) And after all that, someone suffering a catastrophic illness may be left with thousands of dollars in bills from hospitals, physicians, and other health care providers. Many families who thought they had good health insurance have lost their homes and retirement savings because they needed the money to pay medical costs. Also, because the market value of real estate has dropped since 2007, people can no longer rely on home equity loans or home sales to provide income that can be used for medical care.

So the cost of medical care has reached a crisis stage for the elderly and for those approaching retirement. It seems impossible that Medicare and Medicaid will not survive in some form in a wealthy country that spends trillions of dollars on defense, but how will they be paid for? Will deductions from salaries increase greatly? Extending the annual period over which deductions are taken from paychecks would help enormously, according to some analysts. Still, in difficult economic times, with a high level of unemployment, Congress has resisted enacting legislation that will cost workers more in taxes than they pay now.

Although many feel that a single-payer medical system like that in most developed countries would be the best solution to rising health costs for people of all ages, many others oppose that answer. The private insurance companies, for instance, are very powerful and have some influence on legislators' decisions. They have opposed not only a single-payer system but also any public plan for insurance (government payment of part of medical insurance costs).

In the past, Congress was dominated by Republicans, most of whom opposed any change in the current system. Republicans generally oppose any government involvement in health care, and Democrats support at least some role for the government. Since the election of 2008, in which Democrats both won the presidency and became the majority party in Congress, there has been a movement toward establishing some kind of a public plan for people of all ages. This plan would allow those who are ineligible for insurance or who don't have access to coverage to buy coverage at affordable rates through a government-administered plan. Although the elderly already have Medicare, a public plan might help them pay for supplemental insurance. However, many conservatives oppose any government involvement in insurance. The 2010 health plan includes no public plan.

Health care reform has been a major political issue for years, with Democrats like the late Senator Edward Kennedy and President Bill Clinton fighting valiantly but failing to change the system. In the 1930s and 1940s, Presidents Franklin Roosevelt and Harry Truman had also made an effort to help people manage the cost of health care, but the skyrocketing cost in more recent years has focused attention on the problem.

Senator Kennedy died in August 2009 without seeing the changes in health care that were among his major goals. The sadness his death caused in Congress was not sufficient to overcome major opposition to the universal coverage he favored, which was viewed as socialistic by conservatives.

In 2009, both the Senate and the House of Representatives passed bills with the aim of reforming health care, though bitter partisan conflict made it impossible for either bill to become law. Providing popular support for congressional members on the far right, conservative columnists and bloggers accused the president of favoring "death panels" that would "pull the plug on Grandma" to pay for the program. Despite the divisive battle, the House narrowly passed its bill on November 7, and the Senate passed its own on December 24. Senators and representatives began working to merge the two bills, but opposition continued. When a Republican won the special election to fill the late Senator Kennedy's seat, the Democrats lost the 60th vote they needed to block a filibuster by Republicans, and support for reform was threatened further.

President Obama tried for months to influence senators and representatives to come to an agreement. Finally, after summoning many of them to a summit meeting at the White House, he unveiled his own proposal, a compromise that contained elements of both bills. On March 22, 2010, the president signed the Patient Protection and Affordable Care Act (PPACA) into law.

The law will make health insurance coverage mandatory for most Americans, put 16 million more people on Medicaid, and help low- and middle-income citizens by providing subsidies for private insurance coverage. In addition, it will control the actions of private insurers more than has been the case in the past, so that the insurers can no longer deny care for pre-existing conditions or refuse to insure those who have certain conditions. The measure will cost about $938 billion over 10 years; however, the non-partisan Congressional Budget Office has forecast that it will also lower the federal deficit $138 billion over that period. The law satisfies neither political party; conservatives continue their opposition to any involvement of the government in health care, and liberals are unhappy with restrictions on abortions and the lack of a public option for insurance coverage. As this book goes to press in January 2011, the Republicans in Congress are hoping to repeal the law, and its future is uncertain.

For the elderly, the most obvious change will be the gradual elimination of the coverage gap in Medicare Part D. The government's payments to Medicare will lessen, but the president has insisted that this will occur as a result of eliminating waste in the program, not from lowering the standard of care. The expansion in Medicaid enrollees will make that program available to some elderly people who are not yet eligible for Medicare but cannot afford insurance.

One issue that was not addressed in PPACA was the reimbursement of doctors who treat Medicare patients. Because of restrictions on reimbursements and extensive paperwork, many physicians already refuse to accept

Medicare patients. Under current law, Medicare payments to physicians were scheduled to be cut 21% in 2010 (Stolberg, 2010). The president and Congress agreed that it was necessary to forestall the cut, which may lead to even fewer physicians being willing to treat Medicare patients, but there was disagreement on the funding. The Republicans wanted to avoid adding to the deficit, preferring to find a way to pay the billions of dollars that will be needed. Democrats, including Obama, hoped to provide federal funding. In December 2010 Congress passed a bill granting a temporary reprieve for physicians, but it will only last into 2011.

Whatever happens to health insurance in the coming years, it seems inevitable that taxes must increase to cover increased costs of insurance. Although that may be costly and painful, the cost and pain of not doing anything would be far greater in the long run.

MEDICARE

Medicare Part A is an automatic benefit at age 65, with the same amount of free coverage for everyone. It pays a large portion of basic hospital and nursing home costs that are part of inpatient treatment. These costs include a semiprivate room, meals, general nursing, drugs needed for inpatient treatment, and some other hospital services. If medically necessary, Part A pays for part of the cost of a private room. However, the patient must pay separately for private-duty nursing, a telephone, television, and personal care items. (Hospitals are allowed to charge the patient even for small items like razors and slipper socks.) The facilities in which care is provided must be acute care hospitals, critical access hospitals, inpatient rehabilitation facilities, or long-term care hospitals. Also covered are inpatient care as part of a qualifying clinical research study and mental health care. Part A also fully covers blood that the hospital gets from a blood bank. If the hospital must buy the blood, the patient must either pay for the first three units of blood received each calendar year or have the blood donated (by the patient or someone else).

Medicare Part A also covers some home health services, including medically necessary part-time or intermittent skilled nursing care, physical therapy, speech–language pathology, and a continuing need for occupational therapy. The care must be ordered by a doctor, and it must be provided by a Medicare-certified home health agency. These services also may include medical social services, part-time or intermittent home health aide services, durable medical equipment such as wheelchairs and walkers, and medical supplies that will be used at home. To qualify for these home health services, the patient must not be able to leave home without a major effort (must be homebound).

When a patient leaves the hospital after a stay of at least three days, but needs to have daily skilled care such as intravenous injections or physical therapy, Medicare Part A pays for temporary care in a skilled nursing facility. This includes a semiprivate room, meals, skilled nursing and rehabilitative services, and other services and supplies. This benefit does not cover long-term care or custodial care.

Medicare Part B covers nonhospital medical costs, such as doctors' bills, X-rays, and lab tests. Part B also covers the doctor and emergency room services that the patient receives while in a hospital. Unlike Part A, Part B is not free and is optional. However, it covers so many medical costs that about 97% of those who are eligible take advantage of the program (Butler, 1995). The Part B monthly premium for 2010 is a minimum of $96.40 (for individuals whose annual income is $85,000 or less) but may be as much as $308.30, depending on the person's income. The premium is deducted from Social Security payments. If an enrollee fails to sign up for Part B at the same time as Part A, a penalty may be added to payments when the person does enroll in Part B later.

The distinction between copayment (or copays) and coinsurance can be confusing. Usually a copay is a fixed amount, such as $35 for each doctor's visit; coinsurance, in contrast, is a percentage of costs paid by the patient after the annual deductible—the amount that is covered, but is paid by the patient before Medicare pays—has been exceeded. The "You may be billed" column in insurance and Medicare statements may refer to either copays or coinsurance.

Even part of a medical bill can add up to many thousands of dollars, so having a Medigap policy is desirable for paying some of the costs not covered by Parts A and B of Medicare. It is obtained from a secondary insurer and can be purchased only by someone already enrolled in Parts A and B. The secondary insurer is chosen by the individual from a variety of companies such as Blue Cross. Premiums and coverage vary greatly, so it is important to compare the policies carefully before choosing one. Questions to ask before choosing an insurer include:

- What is the monthly premium?
- What copayments are there? Do I have to pay a portion of each bill? If so, how much is the copay?
- What is the annual deductible (the amount I must pay myself each year before coverage begins)?
- Am I eligible for low-income aid that would cover as much as a Medigap policy?

- Is my choice of doctors and other medical providers restricted under the policy?
- How much can the premiums change in the future?
- Is there a waiting period to cover any preexisting conditions?
- Are claims filed electronically to speed payment?

Part C is another name for the Medicare Advantage plan and does not need to concern FFS enrollees. Part D is perhaps the most confusing portion of Medicare, but a good plan is extremely helpful in paying for medicines. An individual chooses a Part D insurer (usually online through the Medicare site) from a large array of companies. Some plans cost very little but provide limited coverage of drugs; others are more expensive and cover all drug costs. Choosing the right plan requires not only knowing what drugs are being taken currently, and in what dosages, but also anticipating likely changes in medication during the next year or so.

Before enrolling in a Part D plan, one should carefully assemble this information:

- All medications needed (preferably listed by both their generic and trade names)
- Dosages of each drug
- Names of local pharmacies
- Names of prescribing doctors

This information is needed for determining which plan is the best for an individual, and having all of it available ahead of time makes the enrollment much simpler. Once enrolled in a Part D plan, it may be difficult to change insurers, so it is important to choose carefully at the beginning.

If even the least costly Plan D plans seem out of reach, a low-income subsidy may help. Social Security will help those who have limited income and resources. Those who are interested can call Social Security at 1-800-772-1213 (or 1-800-325-0778 for TTY users) and ask for form SSA-1020 to find out whether they qualify for extra help in paying for prescription drugs.

November 15 is the annual deadline for signing up for Part D or making changes in coverage. Before that date, people should review their current plan to learn whether any changes are necessary. December 31 is the last day most people can make any changes in Medicare coverage. The handbook *Medicare and You* is mailed (or sent electronically) to all enrollees in October and provides information that should be reviewed carefully. The Web site www.medicare.gov also gives that information. The telephone number for Medicare is 1-800-MEDICARE (1-800-633-4227; 1-877-486-2048 for TTY users).

Medicaid eligibility and benefits vary from state to state. In general, if a person's total assets (other than a home and car) exceed $3,000, as of 2010 they are ineligible for Medicaid.

A 2007 study of Medicare beneficiaries revealed that only 40% realized their Part D plan included a coverage gap, commonly called the "donut hole." After being covered for a certain amount—in many cases, about $2,000— they must pay all their own costs for drugs until they reach a level defined as catastrophic coverage. At that point, they again are covered. There has been much criticism about the way Part D is structured, because those who reach the gap may stop taking needed medicines, reduce the dosages, or be financially burdened (Hsu et al., 2008). The health insurance reform enacted in 2010 includes gradually eliminating the donut hole.

The Obama administration is considering cutting billions of dollars from Medicare and Medicaid, primarily by increasing the programs' efficiency. They believe that these massive cuts to the Medicare and Medicaid programs will be offset by decreasing numbers of uninsured and underinsured patients under proposed new health care legislation that requires everyone to be insured. The argument is that if enough people are insured by private companies, the government will not need to pay the costs of their health care. Some critics argue that the increased private coverage will not be sufficient to protect Medicare funds, because in the current recession consumers cannot afford insurance.

OTHER ISSUES FOR THE ELDERLY

Even those aging people who have insurance may need other kinds of medical-related help. Appropriate housing is always a difficulty. In addition, transportation often becomes a major problem in our automobile-centered society.

Housing

Homes built until about World War II can be difficult for the elderly to live in and maintain. Victorian-era houses, especially, pose problems. Beautiful and prized by many preservationists and homeowners as they still are, the houses have steep stairways, sometimes with no handrails to help those with stiff joints and weakened muscles. Kitchens were poorly planned, even for the more agile, younger servants who did most of the cooking at that time. The carved woodwork is hard to dust and wax, and small panes of glass in windows and doors can be hard to clean. Outdoors, the gingerbread details are costly and difficult to maintain.

The Arts and Crafts homes built at the turn of the 20th century were an improvement from many points of view. Bathrooms were designed for easier cleaning, for instance. The homes included built-in bookcases and china cabinets that were easier to dust and wax. However, their attractive glass windows are hard to clean, like those in Victorian homes. Hardwood floors must be waxed or refinished occasionally. The shingles used on many of the Arts and Crafts homes have cracked and crumbled over the years, which has led to costly repairs. Stairways are steep, and many doorways are narrow. Like Victorian-era homes, they have little insulation; residents must either make costly investments in insulation or resign themselves to being cold in winter and hot in summer.

In the 1920s and 1930s, modern appliances transformed kitchens, and scientific planners designed kitchens for maximum efficiency. The U-shaped kitchen appeared, often featuring all-electric appliances. The homemaker's job became much easier in some respects. Even today, an elderly person might not have too much trouble using a kitchen from that period if the house had only one story.

In many respects, however, the beautiful old homes in which some of the elderly grew up and raised their children are no longer appropriate for people who have heart disease, arthritis, or other difficulties. They may need wide doorways that can accommodate walkers or wheelchairs, electrical outlets and switches at about waist height, grab bars in the bathroom, and faucet handles and doorknobs that can be easily grasped. Bathrooms and bedrooms should be very near each other. Laundry areas should be near kitchens or bathrooms, not in basements. Every room should have a telephone connection. Even a few steps or thresholds may make living in a home difficult for someone who has trouble walking.

To some extent, old homes can be modified for aging residents. A wheelchair ramp can make the house accessible not only for someone using a wheelchair, but also for anyone who has trouble climbing stairs or is pulling a grocery cart. Some who have lived in a home with a ramp have learned to see it as desirable for everyone in the family.

Uksun Kim, an assistant professor of civil and environmental engineering at California State University, Fullerton teaches a class about designing buildings for specific needs; among the buildings are those for aging people. Kim thinks homes should be designed for universal use, so that anyone—including the elderly and the disabled—can live in them comfortably. One part of the design should be partitioned inner walls rather than load-bearing inner walls, so that a home can be remodeled easily for different occupants. Doorways can be widened, closets added or removed, and rooms expanded or divided as necessary.

Planners have been talking about universal design (mainly for people with disabilities) and architecture for the elderly for many years; one would think that the homes built in recent years would have every advantage for older residents. Unfortunately, this is not the case. Apparently unaware that they will not be healthy and vigorous forever, buyers have asked for and gotten large homes with sunken living rooms; slick marble floors; large, elaborate gourmet kitchens; high counters; and other features that are unfriendly to the elderly. Adding insult to injury, the homes with these characteristics are much more expensive than simpler, easier-to-maintain homes. Few of today's elderly could afford new homes, even if they wished to have them.

Fortunately, some older and less expensive houses are still livable. After World War II, the demand for housing for returning veterans and their young families created a demand for large numbers of affordable homes. Developers made sure that towns such as Levittown, Pennsylvania; Park Forest, Illinois; and Daly City, California, sprang up quickly.

The simplest of these stucco-covered homes were built on a single concrete slab; in the final home, the slab was covered with wall-to-wall carpeting, linoleum, or other material. Typically, there were an L-shaped living room/dining room, a large eat-in kitchen, one bathroom, three bedrooms, and a family room. The houses were models of efficiency, often having a combination furnace room/laundry room/utility room in the center. Anyone doing housework could set a roast in the oven, put some laundry in the washing machine or dryer, roll the vacuum cleaner into the next room, and push it around from room to room. The housework, cooking, and laundry were done in record time. The kitchen and family room windows overlooked the backyard, so it was also easy to supervise children playing outdoors. It was an ideal place for a young family.

As the economy improved, many began criticizing these homes. Songwriter Malvina Reynolds, for instance, wrote them off as "ticky-tacky little boxes" that housed people who had no individuality (Reynolds, 1962).

However, for the elderly today, these homes can be lived in longer than more aesthetically pleasing houses. Not only were they easy to clean and maintain, but they have stood the test of time. Owners have added trees and other landscaping, made improvements that made the homes suitable for their individual needs, furnished them attractively, and generally created pleasant living environments. Some of these homes have become expensive as a result, but in general they are still more affordable than houses in many other areas. They are also large enough to house a live-in helper if that becomes necessary, allowing the homeowner to remain home longer than they could without help.

Because they were built before current concerns about the environment, the houses tend to waste energy. Anyone moving into one today may need to add insulation, change windows and doors to conserve energy, and make other changes. Because the houses are small and simply constructed, though, that should not be a major concern.

For some elderly people, apartment living makes sense. Many apartment buildings have wide entrances on the main floor and elevators to other floors, so that climbing stairs is not necessary. (However, those who reside in the buildings are usually required to be mobile enough to climb stairs in an emergency, which is impossible for some people.) Floor plans are usually simple, and housekeeping is easy. No lawn mowing or outdoor maintenance by the tenants is necessary.

Similarly, manufactured houses can be pleasant residences for some elderly people. Some mobile home parks have swimming pools, community centers, and other advantages; some require residents to be aged 55 or more, which appeals to some who prefer having children at a distance.

One major problem with nearly every kind of home is that the resident must leave if his or her mental or physical condition declines greatly. Inevitably, with nearly all homes, there comes a time when a homeowner who has lived long enough must have live-in help or must move to assisted living.

Transportation

In addition to housing, transportation can be a problem nearly everywhere. The elderly person who walks or rides a bicycle for more than a block or two is unfortunately rare. The elderly are more likely to drive (regardless of whether they are competent drivers) or to rely on friends and family to drive where they need to go. The problem is handled best in a city that is large enough to have taxicabs or comfortable vans for the elderly (buses may be a convenient form of travel but often lurch too much for those who are not steady on their feet), but small enough to have shopping and other amenities not too far from residential areas.

Some communities offer free or low-cost transportation for those who cannot drive themselves to medical appointments, but, in many cases, riders must wait a long time to be picked up or may spend hours being driven around a large area where other riders are waiting. If they are already ill, the long wait or ride can make them worse. If public transportation is not satisfactory, family caregivers may be called on to provide transportation for the elderly in addition to their other caregiving responsibilities.

In small towns of the past, an elderly person might be able to walk a couple of blocks to a grocery store, pharmacy, place of worship, or hardware store.

Friends and neighbors might live nearby. There might be a library or movie theater as well. While the destinations in a small town might seem dull or quaint by today's standards, they were at least convenient and accessible.

When should an elderly person stop driving? In many parts of the country, the answer has been "never." People in their 80s and 90s have had or caused well-publicized fatal accidents.

In reaction, younger citizens in some states are calling for legislation that would limit driving privileges by age or test results. In Massachusetts, the legislature is considering changing the laws to increase the amount of testing for elderly drivers. For instance, bill S1929 states that "the registrar shall require that all persons aged 85 or older who are seeking to renew their operator's licenses take a vision and road test before being reissued such license" (Moore, 2010). Bloggers in Boston have angrily noted their observations of elderly drivers who drove too slowly in fast-moving traffic or who nearly struck pedestrians.

The rates of accidents do rise sharply after the age of 70 (Insurance Institute for Highway Safety, 2009), but many critics point out that the criteria for driving should be based on ability rather than age. Obviously, it is simplistic to suggest that no one over the age of 70 is capable of driving safely, or that younger drivers are necessarily better. In fact, it seems likely that younger people are more apt to engage in some of the dangerous behaviors that lead to accidents—talking or texting on cell phones while driving, driving at high speeds, having road rage, and so on. In such cases, they may be skilled drivers whose access to driving can be curtailed only after they have an accident.

Certainly a licensed driver should pass written tests every few years, demonstrate ability behind the wheel, and be physically capable of driving. These basic requirements seem self-evident, and few would argue about them. However, many elderly people continue to drive long after they can do so safely. Even intelligent, competent men and women who function well in other areas of their lives may hold onto their drivers' licenses longer than they should, though they realize the danger to themselves and to others.

Why are they so resistant to behaving sensibly? Because in the United States, it is nearly impossible to live a standard adult life without a car. Perhaps it is easiest in large cities like New York, where there is good public transportation at almost any hour. Even there, though, an elderly person may find it difficult or dangerous to stand at a bus stop for a long time or to compete with other riders for breathing space on a subway. In small towns and rural areas, anyone who cannot drive can quickly become isolated. Friends and relatives can sometimes drive elderly passengers, but that can become burdensome. People in our society do need to drive at least occasionally.

Perhaps in time we will have a solution to the problem. For now, the elderly who want to drive need to take special precautions to drive safely and to keep their licenses. Commonsense suggestions like these can help:

- Do not drive after dark if your vision is limited then or if you are blinded by oncoming headlights.
- Limit your driving to familiar areas where you feel able to handle any situation that is likely to arise. Stay off high-speed interstate highways.
- Drive at the speed limit unless weather disallows it or you must speed up temporarily for safety.
- Take good care of your general health. Good nutrition, exercise, and sleep can help you stay alert. If you feel unwell, don't drive until you feel better.
- Be sure your vision is as good as possible by having cataract surgery if needed and by using good eyeglasses.
- Have your hearing checked, and use hearing aids if necessary.
- Avoid distractions while driving. Ask passengers not to talk if conversation takes your mind off driving.
- Keep your vehicle well maintained at all times. Be sure the windows are clean and free of ice or snow.
- Do not drive under the influence of even small amounts of alcohol or drugs.
- Plan ahead to avoid dangerous intersections, crowded streets around schools, and other places and times that may make driving difficult.
- Have your driving skill checked by a professional instructor, even if your state does not require a driving test for a license. Or take an online self-test such as that at http://www.seniordrivers.org/home/.
- The AARP and some senior centers offer helpful classes in driving techniques. Completing them can even lower insurance costs for some drivers.

An older adult who is no longer able to drive but lives in an area with buses, transit, and other transportation options has the ability to stay mobile well beyond the capacity of many in suburban communities. Affordable, accessible, and suitable housing options can allow older adults to age in place and remain in their community their entire lives. Housing that is convenient to community destinations can provide opportunities for physical activity and social interaction. Communities with a safe and secure pedestrian environment and that are near destinations such as libraries, stores, and places of worship allow older adults to remain independent, active, and engaged.

Combined transportation and land-use planning that offers convenient, accessible alternatives to driving can help older adults reach this goal of an active, healthy lifestyle.

Some medium-sized cities are still good environments for older people. Like small towns, they may have stores, senior centers, and other facilities within walking distance of a person's home. For a retired man or woman who is healthy and interested in lifelong education, living in a college town can be paradise. Libraries, theaters, and museums serve the elderly as well as the student population, and some of them may be accessible by foot or easily managed with public transportation. Lectures at the college may be open to the public. However, living in that kind of environment can be prohibitively expensive for many people.

Large cities were once a good place to grow old, at least for those who could afford to live in safe areas. Neighborhood stores and other amenities had the convenience of a small town but were more sophisticated. Subway trains, streetcars, and buses provided good access to shopping, restaurants, and entertainment. Today, even the wealthy find crime and other urban problems are deterrents to living in large cities; unless people are content to remain in gated areas, they find it difficult to live with freedom. Cities and towns have always posed problems for the elderly. There may be broken sidewalks, no curb cuts for wheelchairs, and other barriers. Recently, architects and city planners have talked about creating an environment that makes life easier for older people, but too little has been done. Public places such as shopping malls are often designed more for young, able-bodied people than for their elders. One can walk for hours on hard, slippery surfaces and see few benches where it is possible to rest for a few minutes. Parks are usually better planned, but in our consumer society, it is much easier to find shopping malls than parks.

Suburban environments are especially difficult for the elderly, because they were planned for younger people who drive to most destinations. The theaters, libraries, and other places elderly people might want to visit are far away. Neighbors no longer drop in for casual visits, even if they live in the same areas. Even walking in a suburban area may be difficult, for there may be no sidewalks, only wide streets designed for commuting drivers. As a result, elderly residents of suburbs are likely to be isolated and lonely.

Some city planners are attempting to modify urban environments for the older population as well as for younger people, to encourage safe pedestrian passage and access to good public transportation. The results have been mixed, however. At present, the best urban environment for many elderly seems to be an old, established neighborhood that still has local stores and other conveniences. Unfortunately, the homes in neighborhoods of that sort may be Victorians or other architectural types with steep stairs and other forbidding details.

Obviously, the growing elderly population will need new kinds of homes and surroundings, where they can be safe without giving up the physical exercise and mental stimulation all people need for health. Architects and land-use planners face many challenges in providing for older citizens as well as for younger adults and for children.

LEGAL ISSUES

Along with creating a will for leaving financial assets to heirs, anyone can benefit from creating a living will and medical power of attorney. These documents protect people from receiving unwanted medical care that may lead, for example, to their being kept in a vegetative state rather than being

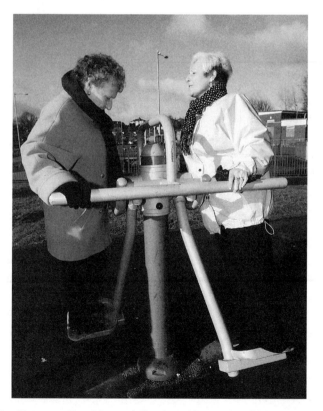

Figure 6.1 Playgrounds with specialized equipment for older people are popular in Europe and Asia. This one is in Manchester, England. (AP Photo/Jon Super.)

allowed to die. Free or low-cost forms are available from many sources on the Internet. Some samples are shown in Appendix A. Many people prefer to pay an attorney to set up these documents (perhaps at the same time that a will is drafted or other legal work is performed), ensuring that they are legal.

The living will is a health care directive, a document that allows a person to give written instructions about medical treatment they do or do not want during a terminal illness. Depending on the person's wishes, a living will can include specific treatments, such as cardiopulmonary resuscitation (CPR), antibiotics, or artificially administered nourishment. In general, medical personnel are legally bound to honor the person's directions. (Parts 2 to 5 of the sample directives in Appendix A correspond to a living will.) The living will takes effect only when the person is too incapacitated to express his or her wishes.

A durable power of attorney for health care gives a trusted person legal authority to act on behalf of an incapacitated person regarding health care decisions. Frank discussion is necessary before the document is signed; the person chosen for this responsibility must have the same views on resuscitation as the person granting the power. Also, the person given the power of attorney must be capable of assertiveness in dealing with medical personnel. In the event of an incapacitating illness, there may be considerable pressure to prolong life by any means, despite the patient's wishes. Legally, the power of attorney must be given access to all medical records and can go to court if necessary to enforce the living will's provisions.

A do-not-resuscitate (DNR) form states that the person who signs it does not want to be resuscitated. It is to be posted in the signer's home where it will be seen by anyone needing to know the person's wishes about not wanting CPR (such as emergency medical technicians who may be called in an emergency). A large DNR label should be added to it.

Living will, DNR, and power of attorney forms vary in different states. It is important to use the approved form for the state in which one lives and to follow state laws about witnesses and notarization. Otherwise, the document is not valid. Copies of these documents should be distributed to all physicians, close relatives, nursing home administrators, clerics, attorneys, and others who may need them. The documents can be revoked at any time, but these people should be notified if they are revoked.

PUBLIC AGENCIES, COMMUNITY RESOURCES

There is an astounding variety of government agencies—federal, state, county, and local—dedicated to the aging. They tend to have good, accessible Web sites, many of which are listed at the end of this book.

Legal help for the elderly is widely available. A local library may have an event when lawyers give pro bono advice, senior centers often have legal departments, and there are some free legal Web sites. Online advice should be followed with great caution; many Web sites are restricted to one state, and some appear to be free but are not.

Libraries also support the elderly in other ways. Like younger people, the elderly can benefit from the millions of free books, films, and other educational and entertaining resources in libraries. In addition, libraries have bulletin boards and racks of information for people of all ages. Most libraries have computers with free access to the Internet. Larger libraries may offer training in computer use.

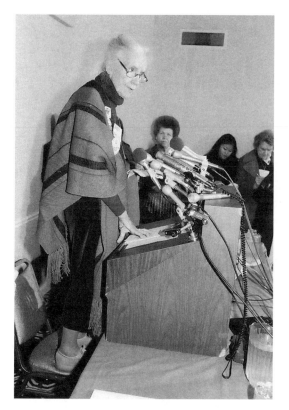

Figure 6.2 Maggie Kuhn at the White House Conference on Aging in Washington, DC, in 1981. The Gray Panthers, the group she founded, aimed to radicalize older Americans and fight the image of the old as useless, infirm, and withdrawn. Once an important political force, the Gray Panthers are now in decline. Sociologists blame the decline on the unwillingness of many over-50 people to think of themselves as aging. (AP Photo/File.)

Senior centers can be a valuable resource for legal and other needs of the elderly. Even in the poorest communities, senior centers are likely to provide helpful advisors and links to public agencies; in wealthy areas, where local residents provide financial support in addition to whatever funds the centers receive from the state, they may have classes, field trips, movies, and other offerings. A senior center director or counselor can help with finding local nursing homes and assisted living residences.

CONCLUSION

Reaching out to others is vital, not a sign of frailty or weakness. By taking advantage of legal and social services, the elderly can empower themselves in many ways. By seeking out good medical providers and following their advice, the elderly can strengthen their bodies and make themselves healthier. Being proactive and independent, yet willing to depend on friends, family, and the larger community, can help the elderly manage their final years as happily and easily as possible.

PART III

References and Resources

Annotated Primary Documents

THE ESTROGEN CONTROVERSY

The following is an abstract of an article published in 2002 that led to major changes in therapy for many postmenopausal women. The results of the study showed that Prempro, a combination of estrogen and progestin, was associated with blood clots, coronary heart disease, and invasive breast cancer.

Risks and Benefits of Estrogen Plus Progestin in Healthy Postmenopausal Women

"Risks and Benefits of Estrogen Plus Progestin in Healthy Postmenopausal Women: Principal Results from the Women's Health Initiative Randomized Controlled Trial." Writing Group for the Women's Health Initiative Investigators. Journal of the American Medical Association. *2002;288: 321–333.*

Context Despite decades of accumulated observational evidence, the balance of risks and benefits for hormone use in healthy postmenopausal women remains uncertain.

Objective To assess the major health benefits and risks of the most commonly used combined hormone preparation in the United States.

Design Estrogen plus progestin component of the Women's Health Initiative, a randomized controlled primary prevention trial (planned duration, 8.5 years) in which 16608 postmenopausal women aged 50–79 years with an intact uterus at baseline were recruited by 40 US clinical centers in 1993–1998.

Interventions Participants received conjugated equine estrogens, 0.625 mg/d, plus medroxyprogesterone acetate, 2.5 mg/d, in 1 tablet (n = 8506) or placebo (n = 8102).

Main Outcomes Measures   The primary outcome was coronary heart disease (CHD) (nonfatal myocardial infarction and CHD death), with invasive breast cancer as the primary adverse outcome. A global index summarizing the balance of risks and benefits included the 2 primary outcomes plus stroke, pulmonary embolism (PE), endometrial cancer, colorectal cancer, hip fracture, and death due to other causes.

Results   On May 31, 2002, after a mean of 5.2 years of follow-up, the data and safety monitoring board recommended stopping the trial of estrogen plus progestin vs. placebo because the test statistic for invasive breast cancer exceeded the stopping boundary for this adverse effect and the global index statistic supported risks exceeding benefits. This report includes data on the major clinical outcomes through April 30, 2002. Estimated hazard ratios (HRs) (nominal 95% confidence intervals [CIs]) were as follows: CHD, 1.29 (1.02–1.63) with 286 cases; breast cancer, 1.26 (1.00–1.59) with 290 cases; stroke, 1.41 (1.07–1.85) with 212 cases; PE, 2.13 (1.39–3.25) with 101 cases; colorectal cancer, 0.63 (0.43–0.92) with 112 cases; endometrial cancer, 0.83 (0.47–1.47) with 47 cases; hip fracture, 0.66 (0.45–0.98) with 106 cases; and death due to other causes, 0.92 (0.74–1.14) with 331 cases. Corresponding HRs (nominal 95% CIs) for composite outcomes were 1.22 (1.09–1.36) for total cardiovascular disease (arterial and venous disease), 1.03 (0.90–1.17) for total cancer, 0.76 (0.69–0.85) for combined fractures, 0.98 (0.82–1.18) for total mortality, and 1.15 (1.03–1.28) for the global index. Absolute excess risks per 10,000 person-years attributable to estrogen plus progestin were 7 more CHD events, 8 more strokes, 8 more PEs, and 8 more invasive breast cancers, while absolute risk reductions per 10,000 person-years were 6 fewer colorectal cancers and 5 fewer hip fractures. The absolute excess risk of events included in the global index was 19 per 10,000 person-years.

Conclusions   Overall health risks exceeded benefits from use of combined estrogen plus progestin for an average 5.2-year follow-up among healthy postmenopausal US women. All-cause mortality was not affected during the trial. The risk-benefit profile found in this trial is not consistent with the requirements for a viable intervention for primary prevention of chronic diseases, and the results indicate that this regimen should not be initiated or continued for primary prevention of CHD.

Writing Group for the Women's Health Initiative Investigators: Jacques E. Rossouw, MBChB, MD, National Heart, Lung, and Blood Institute, Bethesda, Md; Garnet L. Anderson, PhD, Ross L. Prentice, PhD, Andrea Z. LaCroix, PhD, and Charles Kooperberg, PhD, Fred Hutchinson Cancer Research Center, Seattle, Wash; Marcia L. Stefanick, PhD, Stanford University Clinical Center, Stanford, Calif; Rebecca D. Jackson, MD, Ohio State University Clinical Center, Columbus; Shirley A.A. Beresford, PhD, Fred Hutchinson Cancer Research Center, Seattle, Wash; Barbara V. Howard, PhD, MedStar Research Institute, Washington, DC; Karen C. Johnson, MD, MPH, University of Tennessee, Memphis; Jane Morley Kotchen, MD, Medical College of Wisconsin, Milwaukee; Judith Ockene, PhD, University of Massachusetts Medical School, Worcester.

The following is an abstract of an article published in 2006 that brought about a revision in some physicians' recommendations about hormone replacement therapy. It showed that estrogen alone, in contrast to Prempro, a combination of estrogen and progestin, did not increase the risk of breast cancer.

Effects of Conjugated Equine Estrogens on Breast Cancer and Mammography Screening in Postmenopausal Women with Hysterectomy

"Effects of Conjugated Equine Estrogens on Breast Cancer and Mammography Screening in Postmenopausal Women with Hysterectomy." Journal of the American Medical Association. *2006;295: 1647–1657. Copyright © 2006 American Medical Association. All rights reserved.*

Context   The Women's Health Initiative Estrogen-Alone trial comparing conjugated equine estrogens (CEE) with placebo was stopped early because of an increased stroke incidence and no reduction in risk of coronary heart disease. Preliminary results suggesting possible reduction in breast cancers warranted more detailed analysis.

Objective   To determine the effects of CEE on breast cancers and mammographic findings.

Design, Setting, and Participants   Following breast cancer risk assessment, 10,739 postmenopausal women aged 50 to 79 years with prior hysterectomy were randomized to CEE or placebo at 40 US clinical centers from 1993 through 1998. Mammography screenings and clinical breast examinations were performed at baseline and annually. All breast cancers diagnosed through February 29, 2004, are included.

Intervention   A dose of 0.625 mg/d of CEE or an identical-appearing placebo.

Main Outcome Measures   Breast cancer incidence, tumor characteristics, and mammogram findings.

Results   After a mean (SD) follow-up of 7.1 (1.6) years, the invasive breast cancer hazard ratio (HR) for women assigned to CEE vs placebo was 0.80 (95% confidence interval [CI], 0.62–1.04; $P = .09$) with annualized rates of 0.28% (104 cases in the CEE group) and 0.34% (133 cases in the placebo group). In exploratory analyses, ductal carcinomas (HR, 0.71; 95% CI, 0.52–0.99) were reduced in the CEE group vs placebo group; however, the test for interaction by tumor type was not significant ($P = .054$). At 1 year, 9.2% of women in the CEE group had mammograms with abnormalities requiring follow-up vs 5.5% in the placebo group ($P < .001$), a pattern that continued through the trial to reach a cumulative percentage of 36.2% vs 28.1%, respectively ($P < .001$); however, this difference was primarily in assessments requiring short interval follow-up.

Conclusions   Treatment with CEE alone for 7.1 years does not increase breast cancer incidence in postmenopausal women with prior hysterectomy. However, treatment with CEE increases the frequency of mammography screening requiring short interval follow-up. Initiation of CEE should be based on consideration of the individual woman's potential risks and benefits.

Marcia L. Stefanick, PhD; Garnet L. Anderson, PhD; Karen L. Margolis, MD, MPH; Susan L. Hendrix, DO; Rebecca J. Rodabough, MS; Electra D. Paskett, PhD; Dorothy S. Lane, MD, MPH; F. Allan Hubbell, MD, MSPH; Annlouise R. Assaf, PhD; Gloria E. Sarto, MD; Robert S. Schenken, MD; Shagufta Yasmeen, MD; Lawrence Lessin, MD; Rowan T. Chlebowski, MD, PhD; for the WHI Investigators.

THE PROSTATE CANCER CONTROVERSY

The following editorial in the New England Journal of Medicine *summarized the controversy about prostate cancer screening.*

Screening for Prostate Cancer—The Controversy That Refuses to Die
Michael J. Barry, MD

In the United States, most men over the age of 50 years have had a prostate-specific–antigen (PSA) test,[1] despite the absence of evidence from large, randomized trials of a net benefit. Moreover, about 95% of male urologists and 78% of primary care physicians who are 50 years of age or older report that they have had a PSA test themselves,[2] a finding that suggests they are practicing what they preach. And indeed, U.S. death rates from prostate cancer have fallen about 4% per year since 1992, five years after the introduction of PSA testing.[3] Perhaps the answer to the PSA controversy is already staring us in the face. At the same time, practice guidelines cite the unproven benefit of PSA screening, as well as the known side effects,[4,5] which largely reflect the high risks of overdiagnosis and overtreatment that PSA-based screening engenders.[6]

The first reports from two large, randomized trials that many observers hoped would settle the controversy appear in this issue of the *Journal*. In the U.S. Prostate, Lung, Colorectal, and Ovarian (PLCO) Cancer Screening Trial, Andriole et al.[7] report no mortality benefit from combined screening with PSA testing and digital rectal examination during a median follow-up of 11 years.[8] In the European Randomized Study of Screening for Prostate Cancer (ERSPC) trial, Schröder et al.[8] report that PSA screening without digital rectal examination was associated with a 20% relative reduction in the death rate from prostate cancer at a median follow-up of 9 years, with an absolute reduction of about 7 prostate cancer deaths per 10,000 men screened.[8] The designs of the two trials are different and provide complementary insights.

First, one must ask, "Why were these results published now?" Neither set of findings seems definitive; that is, there was neither a clear declaration of futility in the PLCO trial nor an unambiguous net benefit in the ERSPC trial. Both studies are ongoing, with future updates promised. The report on the ERSPC trial follows a third planned interim analysis, which found a marginally significant decrease in prostate-cancer mortality after adjustment of the P value for the two previous looks in an attempt to avoid a false positive conclusion (yet apparently preserving no alpha for the planned final analysis). On the other hand, the investigators in the PLCO trial made the decision to publish their results now because of concern about the emerging evidence of net harm compared with potential benefits associated with PSA screening. Both decisions to publish now can be criticized as premature, leaving clinicians and patients to deal with the ambiguity.

The ERSPC trial is actually a collection of trials in different countries with different eligibility criteria, randomization schemes, and strategies for screening and follow-up. The report by Schröder et al. is based on a predefined core group of men between 55 and 69 years of age at study entry. Subjects were generally screened every 4 years, and 82% were screened at least once. Contamination of the control group with screening as part of usual care is not described. Biopsies were generally recommended for subjects with PSA levels of more than 3.0 ng per milliliter. It is unclear whether the clinicians and hospitals treating patients with prostate cancer differed between the two study groups.

Adjudications of causes of death were made by committees whose members were unaware of study-group assignments, though not of treatments. This point is important, since previous research has suggested that the cause of death is less likely to be attributed to prostate cancer among men receiving attempted curative treatment.[9] Misattribution might then create a bias toward screening, since the diagnosis of more early-stage cancers in the ERSPC trial led to substantially more attempted curative treatments.

The ERSPC interim analysis revealed a 20% reduction in prostate-cancer mortality; the adjusted P value was 0.04. The estimated absolute reduction in prostate-cancer mortality of about 7 deaths per 10,000 men after 9 years of follow-up, if real and not the result of chance or bias, must be weighed against the additional interventions and burdens. The 73,000 men in the screening group underwent more than 17,000 biopsies, undoubtedly many more than did men in the control group, though the latter is not reported. Men had a substantially higher cumulative risk of receiving the diagnosis of prostate cancer in the screening group than in the control group (820 vs. 480 per 10,000 men). Diagnosis led to more treatment, with 277 versus 100 per 10,000 men undergoing radical prostatectomy and 220 versus 123 per 10,000 undergoing radiation therapy with or without hormones, respectively (tentative estimates given the unknown treatments in both groups).

Although estimates of the benefit of screening were somewhat greater for men who actually underwent testing (taking into account noncompliance) than for those who were not tested, the side effects would be proportionately higher as well. Given these trade-offs, the promise of future ERSPC analyses addressing quality of life and cost-effectiveness is welcome indeed. The ERSPC results also reemphasize the need for caution in screening men over the age of 69 years, given an early trend toward higher prostate-cancer mortality with screening in this age subgroup, although this finding may well be due to chance alone.

A final point to make about the ERSPC trial is that to the extent that the diagnosis and treatment of prostate cancer in the screening group differed from those in the control group, it becomes difficult to dissect out the benefit attributable to screening versus improved treatment once prostate cancer was suspected or diagnosed. A similar distribution of treatments among seemingly similar patients with cancer is only partially reassuring in this regard.

Despite a longer median follow-up, the PLCO trial was smaller and therefore less mature than the ERSPC trial, with 174 prostate-cancer deaths driving the power of the study, as compared with 540 such deaths in the ERSPC trial. The screening protocol was homogeneous across sites with an enrollment age of 55 to 74 years and annual PSA tests for 6 years and digital rectal examinations for 4 years, with about 85% compliance. Subjects in the screening group who had a suspicious digital rectal examination or a PSA level of more than 4.0 ng per milliliter received a recommendation for further evaluation. This strategy helped to ensure that any difference in outcome was attributable to screening, rather than downstream management. The effectiveness of screening, of course, will be determined by the effectiveness of subsequent "usual care," but this is the same usual care that many practitioners assume has been responsible for the falling U.S. death rate from prostate cancer. Adjudication of causes of death was similar to that in the ERSPC trial.

Though the PLCO trial has shown no significant effect on prostate-cancer mortality to date, the relatively low number of end points begets a wide confidence interval, which includes at its lower margin the point estimate of effect from the ERSPC trial. Other likely explanations for the negative findings are high levels of prescreening in the PLCO population and contamination of the control group. Contamination was assessed by periodic cross-sectional surveys, with about half the subjects in the control group undergoing PSA testing by year 5. It is unclear whether these estimates reflect testing that year or since trial inception; if the former, the cumulative incidence may be even higher. The smaller difference in screening intensity between the two study groups in the PLCO trial, as compared with the ERSPC trial, is reflected in a smaller risk of overdiagnosis (23% vs. more than 70%) and a less impressive shift in cancer stage and grade distributions. Given that study-group contamination from the use of digital rectal examination was less problematic (only about 25%), ongoing results from both of these trials may necessitate rethinking the role of digital rectal examination in cancer screening.

After digesting these reports, where do we stand regarding the PSA controversy? Serial PSA screening has at best a modest effect on prostate-cancer mortality during the first decade of follow-up. This benefit comes at the cost of substantial overdiagnosis and overtreatment. It is important to remember that the key question is not whether PSA screening is effective but whether it does more good than harm. For this reason, comparisons of the ERSPC estimates of the effectiveness of PSA screening with, for example, the similarly modest effectiveness of breast-cancer screening cannot be made without simultaneously appreciating the much higher risks of overdiagnosis and overtreatment associated with PSA screening.

The report on the ERSPC trial appropriately notes that 1410 men would need to be offered screening and an additional 48 would need to be treated to prevent one prostate-cancer death during a 10-year period, assuming the point estimate is correct. And although the PLCO trial may not have the power as yet to detect a similarly modest benefit of screening, its power is already more than adequate to detect important harm through overdiagnosis. However, the implications of the trade-offs reflected in these data, like beauty, will be in the eye of the beholder. Some well-informed clinicians and patients will still see these trade-offs as favorable; others will see them as unfavorable. As a result, a shared decision-making approach to PSA screening, as recommended by most guidelines, seems more appropriate than ever.

Finally, despite these critiques, both groups of investigators deserve high praise for their persistence and perseverance: to manage such monstrous trials is a herculean task, made no easier when so many observers think the results are self-evident. Further analyses will be needed from these trials, as well as from others—such as the Prostate Cancer Intervention Versus Observation Trial (PIVOT) in the United States (ClinicalTrials.gov number, NCT00007644 [ClinicalTrials.gov])[10] and the Prostate Testing for Cancer and Treatment (PROTECT) trial in the United Kingdom (Current Controlled Trials number, ISRCTN20141297 [controlled-trials.com])[11]—if the PSA controversy is finally to sleep the big sleep.

REFERENCES

1. Ross LE, Berkowitz Z, Ekwueme DU. Use of the prostate-specific antigen test among U.S. men: findings from the 2005 National Health Interview Survey. Cancer Epidemiol Biomarkers Prev 2008;17:636–644.

2. Chan EC, Barry MJ, Vernon SW, Ahn C. Brief report: physicians and their personal prostate cancer-screening practices with prostate-specific antigen: a national survey. J Gen Intern Med 2006;21:257–259.

3. Ries LAG, Melbert D, Krapcho M, et al. SEER cancer statistics review, 1975–2005. Bethesda, MD: National Cancer Institute, 2008.

4. Smith RA, Cokkinides V, Brawley OW. Cancer screening in the United States, 2008: a review of current American Cancer Society guidelines and cancer screening issues. CA Cancer J Clin 2008;58:161–179.

5. U.S. Preventive Services Task Force. Screening for prostate cancer: U.S. Preventive Services Task Force recommendation statement. Ann Intern Med 2008; 149:185–191.

6. Barry MJ. Why are a high overdiagnosis probability and a long lead time for prostate cancer screening so important? J Natl Cancer Inst (in press).

7. Andriole GL, Crawford ED, Grubb RL III, et al. Mortality results from a randomized prostate-cancer screening trial. N Engl J Med 2009;360:1310–1319.

8. Schröder FH, Hugosson J, Roobol MJ, et al. Screening and prostate-cancer mortality in a randomized European study. N Engl J Med 2009;360:1320–1328.

9. Newschaffer CJ, Otani K, McDonald MK, Penberthy LT. Causes of death in elderly prostate cancer patients and in a comparison nonprostate cancer cohort. J Natl Cancer Inst 2000;92:613–621.

10. Wilt TJ, Brawer MK, Barry MJ, et al. The Prostate cancer Intervention Versus Observation Trial: VA/NCI/AHRQ Cooperative Studies Program #407 (PIVOT): design and baseline results of a randomized controlled trial comparing radical prostatectomy to watchful waiting for men with clinically localized prostate cancer. Contemp Clin Trials 2009;30:81–87.

11. Donovan J, Hamdy F, Neal D, et al. Prostate Testing for Cancer and Treatment (ProtecT) feasibility study. Health Technol Assess 2003;7:1–88.

LEGAL ISSUES

The do-it-yourself do-not resuscitate form below is a generic version, provided for illustrative purposes only. It is not a substitute for legal advice. This and similar forms can be found online; many can be downloaded and used without charge. Each state has specific rules about words and content that must be followed for the document to be legal. To be certain that it is legal and up to date, one should consult a local attorney.

Reprinted with permission from the publisher, Nolo Press, Copyright 2010. http://www.nolo.com.

Do-Not-Resuscitate Form

Sample Prehospital Do Not Resuscitate (DNR) Order

Prehospital Do Not Resuscitate (DNR) Order

I, _____ Hector Viera _____ ,
direct that if my heart stops beating or if I stop breathing, no medical procedures be initiated to
resuscitate me, including chest compressions, assisted ventilations, intubation, defibrillation, or
cardiotonic medications.

I hereby agree to and request this Do Not Resuscitate (DNR) order.

If the principal's health care agent or other medical surrogate is signing this form on behalf of the
principal, by signing this form, the surrogate acknowledges that this request to forgo resuscitative
measures is consistent with the known desires of, and with the best interest of, the individual who is the
subject of the form.

Dated: ___February 9, 2009___

Hector Viera
Signature of Principal

Hector Viera
Print Principal's Name

24 Ritter Road
Principal's Address and Phone Number

Calexico, CA 92231

(760) 761-9876

Dated: February 9, 2009

Alicia Machado
Signature of Physician

Alicia Machado
Print Physician's Name

370 E. Birch Street, Suite 205
Physician's Address and Phone Number

Calexico, CA 92231

(760) 761-0123

The do-it-yourself medical power of attorney form below is a generic version, provided for illustrative purposes only. It is not a substitute for legal advice. This and similar forms can be found online; many can be downloaded and used without charge. Each state has specific rules about words and content that must be followed for the document to be legal. To be certain that it is legal and up to date, one should consult a local attorney.

Reprinted with permission from the publisher, Nolo Press, Copyright 2010. http://www.nolo.com.

Medical Power of Attorney Form

Part 1: Power of Attorney for Health Care

(1) **Designation of Agent:** I _____ Chester Larkin _____ , of

16 Deerwood Drive, San Francisco _____ ,

California, designate the following individual as my agent to make health care decisions for me:

Arthur Stimple
Name of Individual You Choose as Agent

16 Deerwood Drive
Address

San Francisco	CA	94114
City	State	Zip Code
(415) 444-5555	(415) 444-1234	
Home Phone	Work Phone	

First Alternate Agent (Optional): If I revoke my agent's authority or if my agent is not willing, able, or reasonably available to make a health care decision for me, I designate as my first alternate agent:

Karen Larkin
Name of Individual You Choose as First Alternate Agent

3421 Euclid Avenue
Address

Berkeley	CA	94709
City	State	Zip Code
(510) 548-5588	(510) 894-4000	
Home Phone	Work Phone	

Second Alternate Agent (Optional): If I revoke the authority of my agent and first alternate agent or if neither is willing, able, or reasonably available to make a health care decision for me, I designate as my second alternate agent:

_____
Name of Individual You Choose as Second Alternate Agent

_____
Address

City	State	Zip Code
Home Phone	Work Phone	

(2) **Agent's Authority:** My agent is authorized to make all health care decisions for me, including decisions to provide, withhold, or withdraw artificial nutrition and hydration and all other forms of health care to keep me alive, except as I state here:

_____
_____
_____
_____

Add Additional Sheets If Needed

(3) **When Agent's Authority Becomes Effective:** My agent's authority becomes effective when my primary physician determines that I am unable to make my own health care decisions unless I mark the following box. If I mark this box ☐ , my agent's authority to make health care decisions for me takes effect immediately.

(4) **Agent's Obligation:** My agent shall make health care decisions for me in accordance with this power of attorney for health care, any instructions I give in Part 2 of this form, and my other wishes to the extent known to my agent. To the extent my wishes are unknown, my agent shall make health care decisions for me in accordance with what my agent determines to be in my best interest. In determining my best interest, my agent shall consider my personal values to the extent known to my agent.

(5) **Agent's Postdeath Authority:** My agent is authorized to make anatomical gifts, authorize an autopsy, and direct disposition of my remains, except as I state here or in Part 3 of this form:

I want my body to be cremated and my ashes to be scattered off the Marin Headlands.

_____

_____

_____

_____

_____

_____

_____

_____

Add Additional Sheets If Needed

(6) **Nomination of Conservator:** If a conservator of my person needs to be appointed for me by a court, I nominate the agent designated in this form. If that agent is not willing, able, or reasonably available to act as conservator, I nominate the alternate agents whom I have named, in the order designated.

Part 2: Instructions for Health Care

If you fill out this part of the form, you may strike any wording you do not want.

(7) **End-of-Life Decisions:** I direct that my health care providers and others involved in my care provide, withhold, or withdraw treatment in accordance with the choice I have marked below:

☒ (a) Choice Not to Prolong Life

I do not want my life to be prolonged if (1) I have an incurable and irreversible condition that will result in my death within a relatively short time, (2) I become unconscious and, to a reasonable degree of medical certainty, I will not regain consciousness, or (3) the likely risks and burdens of treatment would outweigh the expected benefits.

~~☐ (b) Choice to Prolong Life~~

~~I want my life to be prolonged as long as possible within the limits of generally accepted health care standards.~~

(8) **Relief From Pain:** Except as I state in the following space, I direct that treatment for alleviation of pain or discomfort be provided at all times, even if it hastens my death:

_____
_____
_____
_____
_____

Add Additional Sheets If Needed

(9) **Other Wishes:** (If you do not agree with any of the optional choices above and wish to write your own, or if you wish to add to the instructions you have given above, you may do so here.) I direct that:

I do not wish to receive artificial nutrition and hydration under any circumstances except for the treatment of a temporary condition in which I am unable to eat or drink, and then only for a short time. If, within a short time (as determined by my agent after consulting my doctor) there is no benefit to me, then I instruct that artifical nutrition and hydration be withdrawn.

_____

Add Additional Sheets If Needed

Part 3: Donation of Organs at Death

(10) **Wishes for Organ Donation:** Upon my death (mark applicable box):

☒ (a) I give any needed organs, tissues, or parts.

☐ (b) I give the following organs, tissues, or parts only:

_____
_____
_____
_____

Add Additional Sheets If Needed

145

☐ (c) My gift is for the following purposes (strike any of the following you do not want):

    (1) Transplant

    (2) Therapy

    (3) Research

    (4) Education

Part 4: Primary Physician

(11) **Designation of Primary Physician:** I designate the following physician as my primary physician:

Dr. Marcia Silverstein
Name of Physician

555 9th Avenue
Address

San Francisco	CA	94118
City	State	Zip Code

(415) 261-2601
Phone

Secondary Designation: If the physician I have designated above is not willing, able, or reasonably available to act as my primary physician, I designate the following physician as my primary physician:

Name of Physician

Address

City	State	Zip Code

Phone

Part 5: Signatures

(12) **Effect of Copy:** A copy of this form has the same effect as the original.

(13) **Signature:** Sign and date the form here:

Dated: _____December 3, 2008_____

Chester Larkin
Sign Your Name

Chester Larkin
Print Your Name

Alternative #1: Witnesses

(14) **Statement of Witnesses:** I declare under penalty of perjury under the laws of California (1) that the individual who signed or acknowledged this advance health care directive is personally known to me, or that the individual's identity was proven to me by convincing evidence, (2) that the individual signed or acknowledged this advance directive in my presence, (3) that the individual appears to be of sound mind and under no duress, fraud, or undue influence, (4) that I am not a person appointed as agent by this advance directive, and (5) that I am not the individual's health care provider, an employee of the individual's health care provider, the operator of a community care facility, an employee of an operator of a community care facility, the operator of a residential care facility for the elderly, nor an employee of an operator of a residential care facility for the elderly.

First Witness

Chloe Abrams
Signature of Witness

Chloe Abrams
Print Name

2970 16th Street, San Francisco, CA 94103
Address

December 3, 2008
Date

Second Witness

James Lee
Signature of Witness

James Lee
Print Name

849 Valencia Street, San Francisco, CA 94110
Address

December 3, 2008
Date

(15) **Additional Statement of Witnesses:** One of the above witnesses must also sign the following declaration:

I further declare under penalty of perjury under the laws of California that I am not related to the individual executing this advance health care directive by blood, marriage, or adoption, and to the best of my knowledge, I am not entitled to any part of the individual's estate upon his or her death under a will now existing or by operation of law.

James Lee
Signature of Witness

147

Sample Advance Health Care Directive (cont'd)

Alternative #2: Notarization

Certificate of Acknowledgment of Notary Public

State of California

County of _____

} ss

On _____, _____, before me, _____,
personally appeared _____, who
proved to me on the basis of satisfactory evidence to be the person(s) whose name(s) is/are
subscribed to the within instrument and acknowledged to me that he/she/they executed the same
in his/her/their authorized capacity(ies), and that by his/her/their signature(s) on the instrument
the person(s), or the entity upon behalf of which the person(s) acted, executed the instrument.

I certify under PENALTY OF PERJURY under the laws of the State of California that the foregoing
paragraph is true and correct.

WITNESS my hand and official seal.

_____

Notary Public for the State of California

[NOTARY SEAL]   My commission expires _____

(16) **SPECIAL WITNESS REQUIREMENT:** The following statement is required only if you are a patient in a skilled
nursing facility—a health care facility that provides skilled nursing care and supportive care to patients
whose primary need is for availability of skilled nursing care on an extended basis. The patient advocate or
ombudsman must sign the following statement:

Statement of Patient Advocate or Ombudsman

I declare under penalty of perjury under the laws of California that I am a patient advocate or
ombudsman as designated by the State Department of Aging and that I am serving as a witness as
required by Section 4675 of the Probate Code.

_____
Signature of Patient Advocate or Ombudsman

_____
Print Name

_____
Address

_____
Date

SCREENING FOR DEPRESSION

It is important for physicians and caregivers to screen patients for depression by using quick assessment tools. A short form of the Geriatric Depression Scale is shown below. It can be used quickly and easily to assess the likelihood that a person is depressed.

Geriatric Depression Test (short form) (Poon, 1986a)

Instructions to patient:
Circle the answer that best describes how you felt over the past week.

1. Are you basically satisfied with your life?

   yes **no**

2. Have you dropped many of your activities and interests?

   yes no

3. Do you feel that your life is empty?

   yes no

4. Do you often get bored?

   yes no

5. Are you in good spirits most of the time?

   yes **no**

6. Are you afraid that something bad is going to happen to you?

   yes no

7. Do you feel happy most of the time?

   yes **no**

8. Do you often feel helpless?

   yes no

9. Do you prefer to stay at home, rather than going out and doing things?

   yes no

10. Do you feel that you have more problems with memory than most?

    yes no

11. Do you think it is wonderful to be alive now?

    yes **no**

12. Do you feel worthless the way you are now?

    yes no

13. Do you feel full of energy?

    yes **no**

14. Do you feel that your situation is hopeless?

    yes no

15. Do you think that most people are better off than you are?

    yes no

Instructions to physician:
For each **bolded** answer that was circled, score one point.
Total Score _____
A score of 5 or more suggests depression.

HEALTH CARE ISSUES

The following document is President Obama's summary of his compromise health care plan.

Found at http://www.whitehouse.gov/sites/default/files/summary-presidents-proposal.pdf, accessed June 11, 2010.

The President's Proposal February 22, 2010

The President's Proposal puts American families and small business owners in control of their own health care.

- It makes insurance more affordable by providing the largest middle class tax cut for health care in history, reducing premium costs for tens of millions of families and small business owners who are priced out of coverage today. This helps over 31 million Americans afford health care who do not get it today—and makes coverage more affordable for many more.
- It sets up a new competitive health insurance market giving tens of millions of Americans the exact same insurance choices that members of Congress will have.
- It brings greater accountability to health care by laying out commonsense rules of the road to keep premiums down and prevent insurance industry abuses and denial of care.
- It will end discrimination against Americans with pre-existing conditions.
- It puts our budget and economy on a more stable path by reducing the deficit by $100 billion over the next ten years—and about $1 trillion over the second decade—by cutting government overspending and reining in waste, fraud and abuse.

The President's Proposal bridges the gap between the House and Senate bills and includes new provisions to crack down on waste, fraud and abuse It includes a targeted set of changes to the Patient Protection and Affordable Care Act, the Senate-passed health insurance reform bill. The President's Proposal reflects policies from the House-passed bill and the President's priorities. Key changes include:

- Eliminating the Nebraska FMAP provision and providing significant additional Federal financing to all States for the expansion of Medicaid;
- Closing the Medicare prescription drug "donut hole" coverage gap;
- Strengthening the Senate bill's provisions that make insurance affordable for individuals and families;
- Strengthening the provisions to fight fraud, waste, and abuse in Medicare and Medicaid;
- Increasing the threshold for the excise tax on the most expensive health plans from $23,000 for a family plan to $27,500 and starting it in 2018 for all plans;
- Improving insurance protections for consumers and creating a new Health Insurance Rate Authority to provide Federal assistance and oversight to States in conducting reviews of unreasonable rate increases and other unfair practices of insurance plans.

A detailed summary of the provisions included in the President's Plan is set forth below:

Policies to Improve the Affordability and Accountability

Increase Tax Credits for Health Insurance Premiums   Health insurance today often costs too much and covers too little. Lack of affordability leads people to delay care, skip care, rack up large medical bills, or become uninsured. The House and Senate health insurance bills lower premiums through increased competition, oversight, and new accountability standards set by insurance exchanges. The bills also provide tax credits and reduced cost sharing for families with modest income. The President's Proposal improves the affordability of health care by increasing the tax credits for families. Relative to the Senate bill, the President's Proposal lowers premiums for families with income below $44,000 and above $66,000. Relative to the House bill, the proposal makes premiums less expensive for families with income between roughly $55,000 and $88,000. The President's Proposal also improves the cost sharing assistance for individuals and families relative to the Senate bill. Families with income below $55,000 will get extra assistance; the additional funding to insurers will cover between 73 and 94% of their health care costs. It provides the same cost-sharing assistance as the Senate bill for higher-income families and the same assistance as the House bill for families with income from $77,000 to $88,000.

Close the Medicare Prescription Drug "Donut Hole"   The Medicare drug benefit provides vital help to seniors who take prescription drugs, but under current law, it leaves many beneficiaries without assistance when they need it most. Medicare stops paying for prescriptions after the plan and beneficiary have spent $2,830 on prescription drugs, and only starts paying again after out-of-pocket

Table A.1 Tax Credits: Maximum Percent of Income Paid for Premiums

Income for a Family of Four*		House	Senate	President's Proposal
From:	To:			
$22,000	$29,000	1.5%	2.0%	2.0–3.0%
$29,000	$33,000	1.5–3.0%	4.0–4.6%	3.0–4.0%
$33,000	$44,000	3.0–5.5%	4.6–6.3%	4.0–6.3%
$44,000	$55,000	5.5–8.0%	6.3–8.1%	6.3–8.1%
$55,000	$66,000	8.0–10.0%	8.1–9.8%	8.1–9.5%
$66,000	$77,000	10.0–11.0%	9.8%	9.5%
$77,000	$88,000	11.0–12.0%	9.8%	9.5%

*Ranges from 133–150% of poverty, then 150–400% of poverty in 50% increments, rounded to the nearest $1,000

spending hits $4,550. This "donut hole" leaves seniors paying the full cost of expensive medicines, causing many to skip doses or not fill prescriptions at all—harming their health and raising other types of health costs. The Senate bill provides a 50% discount for certain drugs in the donut hole. The House bill fully phases out the donut hole over 10 years. Both bills raise the dollar amount before the donut hole begins by $500 in 2010. Relative to the Senate bill, the President's Proposal fills the "donut hole" entirely. It begins by replacing the $500 increase in the initial coverage limit with a $250 rebate to Medicare beneficiaries who hit the donut hole in 2010. It also closes the donut hole completely by phasing down the coinsurance so it is the standard 25% by 2020 throughout the coverage gap.

Table A.2 Reduced Cost Sharing: Percent of Costs Paid for by Health Insurance Plan

Income for a Family of Four*		House	Senate	President's Proposal
From:	To:			
$29,000	$33,000	97%	90%	94%
$33,000	$44,000	93%	80%	85%
$44,000	$55,000	85%	70%	73%
$55,000	$66,000	78%	70%	70%
$66,000	$77,000	72%	70%	70%
$77,000	$88,000	70%	70%	70%

*Ranges from 133–150% of poverty, then 150–400% of poverty in 50% increments, rounded to the nearest $1,000

Invest in Community Health Centers   Community health centers play a critical role in providing quality care in underserved areas. About 1,250 centers provide care to 20 million people, with an emphasis on preventive and primary care. The Senate bill increases funding to these centers for services by $7 billion and for construction by $1.5 billion over 5 years. The House bill provides $12 billion over the same 5 years. Bridging the difference, the President's Proposal invests $11 billion in these centers.

Strengthen Oversight of Insurance Premium Increases   Both the House and Senate bills include significant reforms to make insurance fair, accessible, and affordable to all people, regardless of pre-existing conditions. One essential policy is "rate review" meaning that health insurers must submit their proposed premium increases to the State authority or Secretary for review. The President's Proposal strengthens this policy by ensuring that, if a rate increase is unreasonable and unjustified, health insurers must lower premiums, provide rebates, or take other actions to make premiums affordable. A new Health Insurance Rate Authority will be created to provide needed oversight at the Federal level and help States determine how rate review will be enforced and monitor insurance market behavior.

Extend Consumer Protections against Health Insurer Practices   The Senate bill includes a "grandfather" policy that allows people who like their current coverage, to keep it. The President's Proposal adds certain important consumer protections to these "grandfathered" plans. Within months of legislation being enacted, it requires plans to cover adult dependents up to age 26, prohibits rescissions, mandates that plans have a stronger appeals process, and requires State insurance authorities to conduct annual rate review, backed up by the oversight of the HHS Secretary. When the exchanges begin in 2014, the President's Proposal adds new protections that prohibit all annual and lifetime limits, ban pre-existing condition exclusions, and prohibit discrimination in favor of highly compensated individuals. Beginning in 2018, the President's Proposal requires "grandfathered" plans to cover proven preventive services with no cost sharing.

Improve Individual Responsibility   All Americans should have affordable health insurance coverage. This helps everyone, both insured and uninsured, by reducing cost shifting, where people with insurance end up covering the inevitable health care costs of the uninsured, and making possible robust health insurance reforms that will curb insurance company abuses and increase the security and stability of health insurance for all Americans. The House and Senate bills require individuals who have affordable options but who choose to remain uninsured to make a payment to offset the cost of care they will inevitably need. The House bill's payment is a percentage of income. The Senate sets the payment as a flat dollar amount or percentage of income, whichever is higher (although not higher than the lowest premium in the area). Both the House and Senate bill provide a low-income exemption, for those individuals with incomes below the tax filing threshold (House) or below the poverty threshold (Senate). The Senate also includes a "hardship" exemption for people who cannot afford insurance, included in the President's Proposal. It protects those who would face premiums of more than 8 percent of their income from having to pay any assessment and they can purchase a low-cost catastrophic plan in the exchange if they choose. The President's Proposal adopts the Senate approach but lowers the flat dollar assessments, and raises the percent of income assessment that individuals pay if they choose not to become insured. Specifically, it lowers the flat dollar amounts from $495 to $325 in 2015 and $750 to $695 in 2016. Subsequent years are indexed to $695 rather than $750, so the flat dollar amounts in later years are lower than the Senate bill as well. The President's Proposal raises the percent of income that is an alternative payment amount from 0.5 to 1.0% in 2014, 1.0 to 2.0% in 2015, and 2.0 to 2.5% for 2016 and subsequent years—the same percent of income as in the House bill, which makes the assessment more progressive. For ease of administration, the President's Proposal changes the payment exemption from the Senate policy (individuals with income below the poverty threshold) to individuals with income below the tax filing threshold (the House policy). In other words, a married couple with income below $18,700 will not have to pay the assessment. The President's Proposal also adopts the Senate's "hardship" exemption.

Strengthen Employer Responsibility   Businesses are strained by the current health insurance system. Health costs eat into their ability to hire workers, invest in and expand their businesses, and compete locally and globally. Like individuals, larger employers should share in the responsibility for finding the solution. Under the Senate bill, there is no mandate for employers to provide health insurance. But as a matter of fairness, the Senate bill requires large employers (i.e., those with more than 50 workers) to make payments only if taxpayers are supporting the health insurance for their workers. The assessment on the employer is $3,000 per full-time worker obtaining tax credits in the exchange if that employer's coverage is unaffordable, or $750 per full-time worker if the employer has a worker obtaining tax credits in the exchange but doesn't offer coverage in the first place. The House bill requires a payroll tax for insurers that do not offer health insurance that meets minimum standards. The tax is 8% generally and phases in for employers with annual payrolls from $500,000 to $750,000; according to the Congressional Budget Office (CBO), the assessment for a firm with average wages of $40,000 would be $3,200 per worker. In other words, a married couple with income below $18,700 will not have to pay the assessment. The President's Proposal also adopts the Senate's "hardship" exemption. Under the President's Proposal, small businesses will receive $40 billion in tax credits to support coverage for their workers beginning this year. Consistent with the Senate bill, small businesses with fewer than 50 workers would be exempt from any employer responsibility policies. The President's Proposal is consistent with the Senate bill in that it does not impose a mandate on employers to offer or provide health insurance, but does require them to help defray the cost if taxpayers are footing the bill for their workers. The President's Proposal improves the transition to the employer responsibility policy for employers with 50 or more workers by subtracting out the first 30 workers from the payment calculation (e.g., a firm with 51 workers that does not offer coverage will pay an amount equal to 51 minus 30, or 21 times the applicable per employee payment amount). It changes the applicable payment amount for firms with more than 50 employees that do not offer coverage to $2,000—an amount that is one-third less than the average House assessment for a typical firm and less than half of the average employer contribution to health insurance in 2009. It applies the same firm-size threshold across the board to all industries. It fully eliminates the assessment for workers in a waiting period, while maintaining the 90-day limit on the length of any waiting period beginning in 2014.

Policies to Crack Down on Waste, Fraud and Abuse   The House and Senate health reform bills contain an unprecedented array of aggressive new authorities to fight waste, fraud and abuse. The President's Proposal builds on those provisions by incorporating a number of additional proposals that are either part of the Administration's FY 2011 Budget Proposal or were included in Republican plans.

Comprehensive Sanctions Database   The President's Proposal establishes a comprehensive Medicare and Medicaid sanctions database, overseen by the HHS Inspector General. This database will provide a central storage location, allowing for law enforcement access to information related to past sanctions on health care providers, suppliers and related entities. (Source: H.R. 3400, "Empowering Patients First Act" (Republican Study Committee bill))

Registration and Background Checks of Billing Agencies and Individuals   In an effort to decrease dishonest billing practices in the Medicare program, the President's Proposal will assist in reducing the number of individuals and agencies with a history of fraudulent activities participating in Federal health care programs. It ensures that entities that bill for Medicare on behalf of providers are in good standing. It also strengthens the Secretary's ability to exclude from Medicare individuals who knowingly submit false or fraudulent claims. (Source: H.R. 3970, "Medical Rights & Reform Act" (Kirk bill))

Expanded Access to the Healthcare Integrity and Protection Data Bank   Increasing access to the health care integrity data bank will improve coordination and information sharing in anti-fraud efforts. The President's Proposal broadens access to the data bank to quality control and peer review organizations and private plans that are involved in furnishing items or services reimbursed by Federal health care program. It includes criminal penalties for misuse. (Source: H.R. 3970, "Medical Rights & Reform Act" (Kirk bill))

Liability of Medicare Administrative Contractors for Claims Submitted by Excluded Providers   In attacking fraud, it is critical to ensure the contractors that are paying claims are doing their utmost to ensure excluded providers do not receive Medicare payments. Therefore, the President's Proposal provision holds Medicare Administrative Contractors accountable for Federal payment for individuals or entities excluded from the Federal programs or items or services for which payment is denied. (Source: H.R. 3970, "Medical Rights & Reform Act" (Kirk bill))

Community Mental Health Centers   The President's Proposal ensures that individuals have access to comprehensive mental health services in the community setting, but strengthens standards for facilities that seek reimbursement as community mental health centers by ensuring these facilities are not taking advantage of Medicare patients or the taxpayers. (Source: H.R. 3970, "Medical Rights & Reform Act" (Kirk bill))

Limiting Debt Discharge in Bankruptcies of Fraudulent Health Care Providers or Suppliers   The President's Proposal will assist in recovering overpayments made to providers and suppliers and return such funds to the Medicare Trust Fund. It prevents fraudulent health care providers from discharging through bankruptcy amounts due to the Secretary from overpayments. (Source: H.R. 3970, "Medical Rights & Reform Act" (Kirk bill))

Use of Technology for Real-Time Data Review   The President's Proposal speeds access to claims data to identify potentially fraudulent payments more quickly. It establishes a system for using technology to provide real-time data analysis of claim and payments under public programs to identify and stop waste, fraud and abuse. (Source: Roskam Amendment offered in House Ways & Means Committee markup)

Illegal Distribution of a Medicare or Medicaid Beneficiary Identification or Billing Privileges   Fraudulent billing to Medicare and Medicaid programs costs taxpayers millions of dollars each year. Individuals looking to gain access to a beneficiary's personal information approach Medicare and Medicaid beneficiaries with false incentives. Many beneficiaries unwittingly give over this personal information without ever receiving promised services. The President's Proposal adds strong sanctions, including jail time, for individuals who purchase, sell or distribute Medicare beneficiary identification numbers or billing privileges under Medicare or Medicaid—if done knowingly, intentionally, and with intent to defraud. (Source: H.R. 3970, "Medical Rights & Reform Act" (Kirk bill))

Study of Universal Product Numbers Claims Forms for Selected Items and Services under the Medicare Program   The President's Proposal requires HHS to study and issue a report to Congress that examines the costs and benefits of assigning universal product numbers (UPNs) to selected items and services reimbursed under Medicare. The report must examine whether UPNs could help improve the efficient operation of Medicare and its ability to detect fraud and abuse. (Source: H.R. 3970, "Medical Rights & Reform Act" (Kirk bill), Roskam Amendment offered in House Ways & Means Committee markup)

Medicaid Prescription Drug Profiling   The President's Proposal requires States to monitor and remediate high-risk billing activity, not limited to prescription drug classes involving a high volume of claims, to improve Medicaid integrity and beneficiary quality of care. States may choose one or more drug classes and must develop or review and update their care plan to reduce utilization and remediate any preventable episodes of care where possible. Requiring States to monitor high-risk billing activity to identify prescribing and utilization patterns that may indicate abuse or excessive prescription drug utilization will assist in improving Medicaid program integrity and save taxpayer dollars. (Source: President's FY 2011 Budget)

Medicare Advantage Risk Adjustment Errors   The President's Proposal requires in statute that the HHS Secretary extrapolate the error rate found in the risk adjustment data validation (RADV) audits to the entire Medicare Advantage contract payment for a given year when recouping overpayments. Extrapolating risk score errors in MA plans is consistent with the methodology used in the Medicare fee-for-service program and enables Medicare to recover risk adjustment overpayments. MA plans have an incentive to report more severe beneficiary diagnoses than are justified because they receive higher payments for higher risk scores. (Source: President's FY 2011 Budget)

Modify Certain Medicare Medical Review Limitations   The Medicare Modernization Act of 2003 placed certain limitations on the type of review that could be conducted by Medicare Administrative Contractors prior to the payment of Medicare Part A and B claims. The President's Proposal modifies these statutory provisions that currently limit random medical review and place statutory limitations on the application of Medicare prepayment review. Modifying certain medical review limitations will give Medicare contractors better and more efficient access to medical records and claims, which helps to reduce waste, fraud and abuse. (Source: President's FY 2011 Budget)

Establish a CMS-IRS Data Match to Identify Fraudulent Providers   The President's Proposal authorizes the Centers for Medicare & Medicaid Services (CMS) to work collaboratively with the Internal Revenue Service (IRS) to determine which providers have seriously delinquent tax debt to help identify potentially fraudulent providers sooner. The data match will primarily target certain high-risk provider types in high-vulnerability areas. This proposal also enables both IRS and Medicare to recoup any monies owed to the Federal government through this program. By requiring the Internal Revenue Service (IRS) to disclose to CMS those entities that have evaded filing taxes and matching the data against provider billing data, this proposal will enable CMS to better detect fraudulent providers billing the Medicare program. (Source: President's FY 2011 Budget)

Preventing Delays in Access to Generic Drugs   Currently, brand-name pharmaceutical companies can delay generic competition through agreements whereby they pay the generic company to keep its drug off the market for a period of time, called "pay-for-delay." This hurts consumers by delaying their access to generic drugs, which are usually less expensive than their branded counterparts. The Federal Trade Commission (FTC) recently estimated that this could cost consumers $35 billion over 10 years. The President's proposal adopts a provision from the bipartisan legislation that gives the FTC enforcement authority to address this problem. Specifically, it makes anti-competitive and unlawful any agreement in which a generic drug manufacturer receives anything of value from a brand-name drug manufacturer that contains a provision in which the generic drug manufacturer agrees to limit or forego research, development, marketing, manufacturing or sales of the generic drug. This presumption can only be overcome if the parties to such an agreement demonstrate by clear and convincing evidence that the pro-competitive benefits of the agreement outweigh the anti-competitive effects of the agreement. The proposal also requires the Chief Executive Officer of the branded pharmaceutical company to certify to the accuracy and completeness of any agreements required to be filed with the FTC.

Policies to Contain Costs and Ensure Fiscal Sustainability

Improve Medicare Advantage Payments   Medicare currently overpays private plans by 14 percent on average to provide the same benefits as the traditional program—and much more in some areas of the country. The Medicare Advantage program has also done little to reward quality. Moreover, plans have gamed the payment system in ways that drive up the public cost of the program. All of this is why Medicare Advantage has become a very profitable line of business for some of the nation's largest health insurers. The Senate bill creates a bidding model for payment rates and phases in changes to limit potential disruptions for beneficiaries. The House proposal phases payments down based on local fee-for-service costs. The President's Proposal represents a compromise between the House and Senate bills, blending elements of both bills, while providing greater certainty of cost savings by linking to current fee-for-service costs. Specifically, the President's Proposal creates a set of benchmark payments at different percentages of the current average fee-for-service costs in an area. It phases these benchmarks in gradually in order to avoid disruption to beneficiaries, taking into account the relative payments to fee-for-service costs in an area. It provides bonuses for quality and enrollee satisfaction. It adjusts rebates of savings between the benchmark payment and actual plan bid to take into account the transition as well as a plan's quality rating: plans with low quality scores receive lower rebates (i.e., can keep less of any savings they generate). Finally, the President's Proposal requires a payment adjustment for unjustified coding patterns in Medicare Advantage plans that have raised payments more rapidly than the evidence of their enrollees' health status and costs suggests is warranted, based on actuarial analysis. This is the primary source of additional savings compared to the Senate proposal.

Delay and Reform the High-Cost Plan Excise Tax   Part of the reason for high and rising insurance costs is that insurers have little incentive to lower their premiums. The Senate bill includes a tax on high-cost health insurance plans. CBO has estimated that this policy will reduce premiums as well as contribute to long-run deficit reduction. The President's Proposal changes the effective date of the Senate policy from 2013 to 2018 to provide additional transition time for high-cost plans to become more efficient. It also raises the amount of premiums that are exempt from the assessment from $8,500 for singles to $10,200 and from $23,000 for families to $27,500 and indexes these amounts for subsequent years at general inflation plus 1 percent. To the degree that health costs rise unexpectedly quickly between now and 2018, the initial threshold would be adjusted upwards automatically. To ensure that the tax affects firms equitably, the President's Proposal reforms it by including an adjustment for firms whose health costs are higher due to the age or gender of their workers, and by no longer counting dental and vision benefits as potentially taxable benefits. The President's Proposal maintains the Senate bill's permanent adjustment in favor of high-risk occupations such as "first responders."

Broaden the Medicare Hospital Insurance (HI) Tax Base for High-Income Taxpayers   Under current law, people who earn a salary pay the Medicare HI tax on their earned income, but those who have substantial unearned income do not, raising issues of fairness. The House bill includes a 5.4% surcharge on high-income households to improve the fairness of the tax system and to support health reform. The Senate bill includes an increase in the HI tax for high-income households for similar reasons, an increase of 0.9% on earnings above a specific threshold for a total employee assessment of 2.35% on these amounts. The President's Proposal adopts the Senate bill approach and adds a 2.9 percent assessment (equal to the combined employer and employee share of the existing HI tax) on income from interest, dividends, annuities, royalties and rents, other than such income which is derived in the ordinary course of a trade or business which is not a passive activity (e.g., income from active participation in S corporations) on taxpayers with respect to income above $200,000 for singles and $250,000 for married couples filing jointly. The additional revenues from the tax on earned income would be credited to the HI trust fund and the revenues from the tax on unearned income would be credited to the Supplemental Medical Insurance (SMI) trust fund.

Increase in Fees on Brand Name Pharmaceuticals   As more Americans gain health insurance, more will be able to pay for prescription drugs. Moreover, the President's plan closes the Medicare "donut hole," ensuring that seniors do not skip or cut back on needed prescriptions. Both policies will result in new revenue for the pharmaceutical industry. The President's Proposal increases the revenue from the assessment on this industry which is $23 billion in the Senate bill by $10 billion over 10 years. It also delays the implementation of these fees by one year, until 2011, and makes changes to facilitate administration by the IRS.

Close Tax Loopholes   Adopts two House proposals to close tax loopholes: (1) Current law provides a tax credit for the production of cellulosic biofuels. The credit was designed to promote the production and use of renewable fuels. Certain liquid byproducts derived from processing paper or pulp (known as "black liquor" when derived from the kraft process) were not intended to be covered by this credit. The President's Proposal adopts the House bill's policy to clarify that they are not eligible for the tax credit. (2) The President's Proposal helps prevent unjustified tax shelters by clarifying the circumstances under which transactions have "economic substance" (as opposed to being undertaken solely to obtain tax benefits) and raises the penalties for transactions that lack economic substance. In so doing, it adopts the House's policy, with minor technical changes.

Other Policy Improvements

Improve the Fairness of Federal Funding for States   States have been partners with the Federal government in creating a health care safety net for low-income and vulnerable populations. They administer and share in the cost of Medicaid and the Children's Health Insurance Program (CHIP). The Senate bill creates a nationwide Medicaid eligibility floor as a foundation for exchanges at $29,000 for a family of 4 (133% of poverty)—and provides financial support that varies by State to do so. Relative to the Senate bill, the President's Proposal replaces the variable State support in the Senate bill with uniform 100% Federal support for all States for newly eligible individuals from 2014 through 2017, 95%

support for 2018 and 2019, and 90% for 2020 and subsequent years. This approach resembles that in the House bill, which provided full support for all States for the first two years, and then 91% support thereafter. The President's Proposal also recognizes the early investment that some States have made in helping the uninsured by expanding Medicaid to adults with income below 100% of poverty by increasing those States' matching rate on certain health care services by 8 percentage points beginning in 2014. The President's Proposal also provides additional assistance to the Territories, raising the Medicaid funding cap by 35% rather than the Senate bill's 30%.

Simplify Income Definitions   The President's Proposal seeks to simplify eligibility rules for various existing programs as well as for the new tax credits. Consistent with some of the policies in the House bill, the President's Proposal will conform income definitions to make the system simpler for beneficiaries to navigate and States and the Federal government to administer by: changing the definition of income used for assistance from modified gross income to modified adjusted gross income, which is easier to implement; creating a 5% income disregard for certain Medicaid eligibility determinations to ease the transition from States' current use of income disregards; streamlining the income reconciliation process for determining tax credits and reduced cost sharing; and clarifying the tax treatment of employer contributions for adult dependent coverage.

Delay and Reform of Fees on Health Insurance Providers   Like the drug industry, the health insurance industry stands to gain as more Americans get coverage. The Senate bill includes a $67 billion assessment on health insurers over 10 years to offset some of the cost of enrolling millions of Americans in their plans. The President's Proposal delays the assessment until 2014 to coincide with broader coverage provisions which will substantially expand the market for health insurance providers. It provides limited exemptions for plans that serve critical purposes for the community, including non-profits that receive more than 80 percent of their income from government programs targeting low-income or elderly populations, or those with disabilities, as well as for voluntary employees' beneficiary associations (VEBAs) that are not established by employers.

Delay and Convert Fee on Medical Device Manufacturers to Excise Tax   The medical device industry also stands to gain from expanding health insurance coverage. Both the House and Senate bills raise $20 billion in revenue from this industry over 10 years. The President's Proposal replaces the medical device fee with an excise tax (yielding the same revenue) that starts in 2013 to facilitate administration by the IRS.

Strengthen the CLASS Act   The House and Senate health insurance reform proposals include the Community Living Assistance Services and Supports (CLASS) Program, a voluntary, privately-funded long-term services insurance program. The CLASS Program offers workers an optional payroll deduction for an insurance program that provides a cash benefit if they become disabled. The President's Proposal makes a series of changes to the Senate bill to improve the CLASS program's financial stability and ensure its long-run solvency.

Protect the Social Security Trust Funds The President's Proposal provides that, if necessary, funds will be transferred to the Social Security Trust Funds to ensure that they are held harmless by the Proposal.

Ensure Effective Implementation The policy changes in health insurance reform will require careful, effective, deliberate, and transparent implementation. The President's Proposal appropriates $1 billion for the Administration to implement health insurance reform policies. It also delays several of the policies to ensure effective implementation and improve transitions: the therapeutic discovery credit, elimination of the deduction for expenses allocable to the Medicare Part D subsidy, the pharmaceutical and medical device industry fees, and the health insurance industry fee.

APPENDIX B

Timeline

1906	Alzheimer's disease first described by German neurologist Alois Alzheimer
1914	Publication of *Geriatrics: The Diseases of Old Age and Their Treatment,* by Ignatz Nascher, who coined the term *geriatrics*
1929	Beginning of the Great Depression, leading to private health insurance that excluded payments for chronic care
1935	Passage of Social Security Act, providing a source of funds for nursing homes
1942	American Geriatrics Society founded
1945	Gerontological Society of America founded
1950	White House Conferences on Aging begun, advancing national initiatives on medical and other problems of the aging
1953	*Journal of the American Geriatrics Society* founded
1965	Passage of Medicare and Medicaid, providing financial help for elderly and disabled patients; Older Americans Act passed, for developing social services
Mid-1960s	Rising role of nurse practitioners in response to national shortage of physicians
1974	National Institute on Aging founded
1980	Hemlock Society formed, advocating the right to die
1980s	Enrollment of many Medicare beneficiaries in health maintenance organizations
1982	Beginning of Women's Health Initiative study by the National Institutes of Health
1988	First examination in geriatric medicine, with passing candidates awarded the Certificate of Added Qualifications in geriatric medicine

1996   Alliance for Aging Research submitted report to United States
               Senate that documented the shortage of physicians with training
               in geriatrics
1999   Jack Kevorkian sentenced to prison for murder after showing a
               video of a patient's death by injection on television (released on
               parole in 2007)
2008   Global recession threatens cuts in medical programs
2009   President Obama proposes reforms in health programs, mainly
               supported by Democrats and opposed by Republicans. Senate
               and House bills passed at the end of the year
2010   President's compromise health plan approved by narrow margin
               in Congress, with provisions that were only partly satisfactory
               to each political party

APPENDIX C

Web Sites

Table C.1

Topic	Sponsor	URL	Comments
History of geriatrics			
	American Geriatrics Society	http://www.americangeriatrics.org/	Official Web site of the American Geriatrics Society
	British Geriatrics Society	http://www.bgs.org.uk/	Official Web site of the British Geriatrics Society
	Canadian Geriatrics Society	http://www.canadiangeriatrics.com/	Official Web site of the Canadian Geriatrics Society
Agencies			
	National Center on Elder Abuse (NCEA)	http://www.ncea.aoa.gov	Directed by the U.S. Administration on Aging, the NCEA is a resource for policy-makers, practitioners, and the public
	Medicare	http://www.medicare.gov	Official government Medicare site
	U.S. Department of Health and Human Services	http://www.cms.hhs.gov	Centers for Medicaid & Medicare Services (a division of the U.S. Department of Health and Human Services); provides rules, forms, and guidance

Medical resources			
	PubMed online	http://www.ncbi.nlm.nih.gov/pubmed/	Site from which medical journals can be searched
	Medline	http://www.nlm.nih.gov/medlineplus/	Medical information in layperson's terms
	National Institute on Aging and the National Library of Medicine	http://www.nihsenior health.gov	Health information for seniors, in type that can be enlarged
	National Osteoporosis Foundation	http://www.nof.org	Information about osteoporosis
	National Eye Institute, National Institutes of Health	http://www.nei.nih.gov	Information about the eyes
	Kaiser Family Foundation	http://www.kff.org	Health information for the public
	New York Times (health section)	http://www.nytimes.com/pages/health	Current news about medical research; especially informative on Tuesdays
	Mayo Clinic	http://www.mayoclinic.com/health/hearing-loss	Information on hearing loss causes and treatment
	National Institutes of Health	http://druginfo.nlm.nih.gov/drugportal/drugportal.jsp	Information on drugs, actions, and side effects
	National Institutes of Health	http://www.nih.gov	Medical research results and general health information

(Continued)

Table C.1 (*Continued*)

Topic	Sponsor	URL	Comments
	National Institute on Mental Health	http://www.nimh.nih.gov/health/topics/older-adults-and-mental-health/index.shtml	Older adults and mental health
	Alcoholics Anonymous	http://www.aa.org	Support group for alcoholics
	LifeRing	http://www.unhooked.com	Support group for alcoholics
	Centers for Disease Control and Prevention	http://www.cdc.gov/	Information on infectious diseases, vaccinations, and health
	Merck & Co., Inc.	http://www.merck.com/mkgr/mmg/home.jsp	Online *Merck Manual of Geriatrics*
	Mayo Clinic	http://www.mayoclinic.com/	Medical information and tools for health
	National Institutes of Health	http://www.cancer.gov/bcrisktool/	Risk-assessment tool for breast cancer
	Alzheimer's Association	http://www.alz.org	Information about Alzheimer's disease
	National Institute of Dental and Craniofacial Research	http://www.nidcr.nih.gov	Information about oral health
	American Dental Association	http://www.ada.org	Professional association for dentists
	National Institute on Aging and the National Library of Medicine	http://www.nihseniorhealth.gov	Health information for older adults

	National Institute on Aging Information Center	http://www.nia.nih.gov	Information about aging and health
	Journal of the American Medical Association	http://www.jama.ama-assn.org/	Professional journal for physicians
Safety	AAA Foundation for Traffic Safety	http://www.seniordrivers.org/home/.	Information and self-tests to help drivers
	National Highway Traffic Safety Organization	http://www.nhtsa.dot.gov/portal/site/nhtsa/menuitem.31176b9b03647a189ca8e410dba046a0/	Older Drivers Program
	National Association of Area Agencies on Aging	http://www.n4a.org/older_driver_safety/materials.cfm	Older Driver Safety Project
Social topics	Federal Trade Commission	http://www ftc.gov	Information for consumers about fraudulent practices in relation to funerals and other purchases
Caregiving	National Alliance for Caregiving	http://www.caregiving.org/data/CaregivingUSAllAgesExecSum.pdf	Caregiving statistics
	National Association of Professional Geriatric Care Managers	http://www.caremanager.org/	Finding a geriatric care manager

(Continued)

Table C.1 (*Continued*)

Topic	Sponsor	URL	Comments
Psychology of aging			
	American Psychological Association (APA)	http://www.apa.org/pi/aging	APA Office on Aging
	American Psychological Association	http://www.apa.org/practice/guidelines/adult.pdf	Guidelines for professionals working with older adults
Legal sites			
	Nolo Press	http://www.nolo.com/	Legal information for the public; do-it-yourself legal forms
	National Academy of Elder Law Attorneys	http://www.naela.com/	Attorneys specializing in elder law
	American Bar Association (ABA)	http://www.abanet.org/aging	ABA Commission on Law and Aging
Housing			
	Cohousing Association of the United States	http://www.cohousing.org	Information about cohousing; directory of homes
General			
	Benefits Check Up	http://www.benefitscheckup.org/	Service that screens for benefits programs for older adults
	U.S. Department of Veterans Affairs	http://www.va.gov	Information for veterans

American Association of Retired Persons (AARP)	http://www.aarp.org/	Official Web site of AARP
Public Health Portal of the European Union	http://ec.europa.eu/health-eu/my_health/elderly/index_en.htm	Geriatric care in the European Union
Administration on Aging	http://www.aoa.gov/eldfam/How_To_Find/How_To_Find.asph	How to find help about aging
National Disability Rights Network	http://www.napas.org/	Help for the disabled
National Association of Area Agencies on Aging	http://www.n4a.org/	Umbrella organization for local agencies dealing with aging
National Council on Aging	http://www.ncoa.org	Web site for the National Council on Aging
Administration on Aging	http://www.aoa.gov/prof/prof.asp	Aging information for professionals

GLOSSARY

Acetylcholine   A chemical that helps to send many signals across synapses to neurons that store memories.

Acetylcholinesterase (ACE) inhibitor   A drug that inhibits the breakdown of acetylcholine.

Activities of daily living (ADLs)   Bathing, dressing, toileting, taking medicines, feeding, and so on. The ability of a person to carry out ADLs is used to assess the level of care needed.

Advance health care directive   A living will.

Aerobic exercise   Exercise that increases the rate of metabolism by increasing oxygen consumption.

Albumin   A simple protein found in the blood.

Alkaline phosphatase   An enzyme found in the liver and kidneys.

Alzheimer's disease   The most common form of dementia. Alzheimer's disease is a degenerative brain disease of unknown cause that usually appears in late middle age or in old age. It is characterized at the tissue level by the degeneration of brain neurons and by tangles and plaques containing beta-amyloid, a protein product.

Amyloid   A substance consisting mainly of protein, which accumulates on neurons in patients with Alzheimer's disease.

Anaerobic exercise   Exercise that builds muscle mass without increasing oxygen consumption.

Anesthesiologist   Physician who gives a patient an anesthetic before or during surgery.

Aneurysm   Ballooning of a blood vessel, forming a blood-filled bulge.

Angina pectoris   Often called angina. Chest pain resulting from too little oxygen reaching the heart muscle.

Angioplasty   Surgical clearing of a blood vessel.

Antioxidant   Compound that opposes the oxidation that damages plant or animal cells. Many brightly colored fruits and vegetables have an antioxidant effect.

Apnea   Temporary lack of breathing during sleep.

Apoplexy   Stroke.

Arrhythmia   An alteration in the force or rate of the heartbeat, or palpitations.

Atherosclerosis   Commonly called hardening of the arteries. Caused by the deposition of fatty plaques in the arteries.

Attending physician   Physician in a teaching hospital who has the overall responsibility for a patient's care and treatment.

Auricles   Upper chambers of the heart.

Autoimmune diseases   Diseases resulting from the body's reacting to itself as if to a foreign protein. Autoimmune diseases include type 1 diabetes and rheumatoid arthritis.

Axon   The part of a neuron that transmits an impulse to the next neuron in a series.

Balloon angioplasty   Widening of a blood vessel with a balloonlike device.

Bilirubin   A pigment found in bile and blood.

Bipolar disorder   A mental disorder usually characterized by mood swings from mania to depression.

Blepharitis   Inflammation of the eyelids.

Blood urea nitrogen   Nitrogen from urea that is found in the blood.

Body mass index   An indication of weight status, determined by a formula that includes height and weight.

Bradykinesia   Abnormally slow movement; characteristic of Parkinson's disease, especially.

BRCA1 and BRCA2 genes   Genes that increase the risk of breast and ovarian cancer.

Cachexia   Physical wasting, usually from malnutrition.

Carcinoma   Cancer.

Cardiovascular disease   Any disease of the circulatory system, including hypertension, atherosclerosis, and heart failure.

Cataract   A cloudiness of the lens of an eye, resulting in decreased vision.

Catarrh   Inflammation of the mucous membranes.

Centers for Disease Control and Prevention   The government agency that maintains and distributes information about disease.

Cerebrovascular disease   Disease in the cerebral part of the brain and the blood vessels associated with it.

Certified nursing assistant   A nursing assistant who performs much of the day-to-day patient care, such as bathing, toileting, and lifting patients.

Charge nurse   The nurse who is the supervisor of nursing during each shift in a hospital or nursing home. Responsible for overseeing patient care during that shift and for working with patients and their families as necessary.

Cholesterol   Steroid found in many body tissues. As a component of low-density lipoproteins, an elevated level of cholesterol may lead to atherosclerosis.

Chronic obstructive pulmonary disease   Chronic bronchitis, emphysema, asthma, and other chronic respiratory diseases.

Claudication   Leg cramps or tiredness resulting from poor circulation.

Colonoscopy   An examination of the entire colon and rectum.

Computed tomography (CT) scan   Often called a cat scan. Radiography resulting in a three-dimensional image of a body structure. The image is constructed from a series of cross-sectional images made along one axis of the structure.

Continuous positive air pressure   A device that pushes air into the lungs during sleep, making normal breathing and sleeping possible for people with apnea.

Cornea   The transparent outer coat of the eye.

Coronary bypass   A surgical procedure that redirects the flow of blood around damaged coronary (heart) blood vessels to make normal circulation to the heart muscle possible.

Creatine   A nitrogenous substance in the muscles.

Creatinine   A nitrogenous substance formed from creatine and found in the urine and blood.

Dementia   A progressive deterioration of the mind. Dementia may be caused by Alzheimer's disease or other disorders.

Diabetes, type 1   The disease resulting from a complete lack of the hormone insulin. This was formerly known as juvenile diabetes.

Diabetes, type 2   The disease resulting from a deficiency of the hormone insulin. This was formerly known as adult-onset diabetes.

Dialysis   Removal of toxins from the blood by an artificial kidney that passes the blood through semipermeable membranes and returns the purified blood to the body.

Diastolic blood pressure   The pressure exerted on blood vessel walls when the heart relaxes; the lower number in the blood pressure ratio.

Digital exam   An examination with a gloved finger, usually of the rectum.

Do-not-resuscitate (DNR) order   A direction to emergency personnel stating that a person does not want cardiopulmonary resuscitation or other procedures that may be specified.

Drop attack   A sudden giving way of the legs, causing a person to fall without losing consciousness.

Elderly   A variable adjective to describe older people, usually defined as 65 years or more.

Electrocardiogram   An electrical device that measures heart rate and rhythm.

Employer mandate   A requirement that employers, or at least employers of a certain size, offer coverage to their workers and pay a specified portion of the costs.

Endocarditis   Inflammation of the valves and lining of the heart.

Endocrinologist   Physician who specializes in diseases of the endocrine system; often treats diabetes and other metabolic disorders.

End-stage renal disease   Advanced stage of loss of kidney function, requiring dialysis.

Epidermis   The outer layer of the skin.

Essential tremor   A tremor that appears like Parkinson's but is a different disorder.

Fecal occult blood test   Test for hidden blood in the feces.

Fibroadenomas   Lumps that arise from an overgrowth of connective and glandular tissue in the breast.

Fibrocystic breast disease   Disease causing a blockage in the breast ducts, leading to a buildup of fluid.

Gastroenterologist   Physician who specializes in diseases of the digestive tract.

Geriatrician   Physician who specializes in treating the elderly.

Geriatrics   Branch of medicine that deals with the health and diseases of the elderly.

Gerontology   "The study of old men," literally; research underlying geriatrics.

Globulin   A protein found in the blood and other tissues.

Guaranteed issue   A requirement that health insurers offer coverage to all applicants, regardless of their health status. This ensures that people are not denied coverage due to preexisting conditions or other reasons.

Health cooperatives, or co-ops   Nonprofit, consumer-run entities through which people could buy low-cost health insurance.

Health information technology   The computerized systems and technologies that enable health care organizations to store and share medical information electronically.

Health insurance exchange or connector   A clearinghouse through which individuals, small employers, and others could buy private health insurance at an affordable rate. The exchange could be run by state, regional, or national commissions, which could set benefit standards and establish rules for insurers.

Hematologist   Physician who specializes in diseases and functions of blood.

Homocysteine   A protein found in the blood. High levels are associated with cardiovascular disease and Alzheimer's disease.

Hormone-dependent breast cancer   Cancer in which estrogen can promote the growth of the cancer cells.

Hormone replacement therapy   The use of estrogen (and sometimes progesterone) to treat the symptoms of menopause. Estrogen also reduces the risk of colon cancer and hip fractures.

Hyperglycemia   Abnormally high level of glucose in the blood.

Hyperkalemia   Too high a level of potassium in the blood.

Hypertension   High blood pressure.

Hypertrophy   Overgrowth.

Hypogonadism   Underdeveloped sexual organs resulting from too low a level of testosterone.

Hypotension, postural   A drop in blood pressure that occurs when a person sits or stands suddenly.

Individual mandate   A requirement that individuals obtain insurance coverage.

Infective endocarditis   Infection of the tissue lining the heart.

Intraocular   Inside the eye.

Invasive surgery Surgery involving incision or insertion of an instrument into the body.

Ischemia Lack of blood flow to an organ (such as the heart or brain), caused by blockage of an artery.

Lewy bodies Abnormalities in brain tissue that are seen in small areas in patients with Parkinson's disease, and throughout the brain in patients with Alzheimer's disease.

Licensed vocational nurse or licensed practical nurse Nurse who works under the supervision of a registered nurse or physician. Most can draw blood and measure blood pressure.

Lipoproteins Substances that contain lipids and proteins. Low-density lipoproteins can accumulate in the blood, form plaques, and lead to atherosclerosis.

Living will A document that gives directions about health care in case the signer cannot make decisions and names a medical power of attorney.

Lumpectomy Mastectomy in which surgery is limited to the tumor and some surrounding tissue.

Medical power of attorney A document naming an agent who can speak for the document signer in case the signer is unable to speak or is otherwise unable to express his or her wishes about health care.

Medicare Part A An automatic benefit at age 65, with the same amount of free coverage for everyone. It pays a large part of hospital costs.

Medicare Part B An optional program purchased by Medicare recipients. It pays for a large part of nonhospital costs, such as X-rays, laboratory tests, and physicians' fees.

Medicare Part C A Medicare Advantage plan.

Medicare Part D An optional part of Medicare that pays for a large part of a person's prescribed medicines. It is purchased through a private insurer.

Medigap Insurance policy to supplement Medicare coverage, obtained from a secondary insurer.

Mediterranean-type diet A diet high in fish and plant foods, such as legumes, cereals, fruits, and nuts, and including olive oil and a small amount of wine; it is also low in poultry and red meat. The name comes from the similarity to foods typically eaten in Mediterranean countries.

Melanoma Cancer of the pigment-making cells in the skin; the most serious type of skin cancer.

Metabolic syndrome A complex condition that includes high blood pressure, body fat concentrated around the waist, high cholesterol level, and hyperglycemia.

Micturition   Urination.

Myocardial infarction   Heart attack.

Nephritis   Inflammation of the kidneys.

Nephrologist   Physician who specializes in diseases and functions of the kidneys.

Nephrosis   A noninflammatory kidney disease.

Nephrotic syndrome   Kidney condition characterized by a deficiency of albumin in the blood and its excretion in the urine.

Neurologist   Physician who specializes in diseases and functions of the brain and spinal cord.

Neuron   Brain cell.

Neuropathy   Degeneration of the nerves.

Neurotransmitter   A substance that carries nerve impulses across synapses.

Nocturia   Nighttime urination.

Nonsteroidal anti-inflammatory drugs   Drugs such as aspirin and acetaminophen, which alleviate pain but do not contain steroids.

Nurse practitioner (NP)   A registered nurse who usually also has a master's or doctor's degree and can provide midlevel medical care. In some states, NPs act as primary health care providers.

Oncologist   Physician who specializes in cancer.

Osteoarthritis   Arthritis that results when bony surfaces in the joints are worn down and new bone grows laterally.

Osteoblasts   Bone-forming cells.

Osteoclasts   Bone-resorbing cells.

Osteomalacia   Softening of the bones; an adult disease that is much like rickets in children.

Osteopenia   An early stage of osteoporosis, with some decrease in bone mass.

Osteoporosis   Decreased bone mass, with resulting fragility.

Otoacoustic   Sounds produced by the ears in response to stimulation.

Otoscope   An instrument used to examine the outer ear and the eardrum.

Ovariectomy   Removal of the ovaries.

Over-the-counter medications   Drugs that can be bought without a prescription.

Palliative   Providing comfort and relief from pain without prolonging life.

Parkinson's disease   A chronic progressive neurological disease, usually beginning in later life, marked by tremor of resting muscles, rigidity, slowness of movement, a shuffling gait, and impaired balance.

Pay or play   In health care, this typically refers to the quid pro quo concept in which employers would be required to offer health coverage to their employees or pay into a pool that would provide coverage.

Periodic limb movement disorder   A condition that makes people jerk and kick their legs often during sleep.

Peyronie's disease   A condition marked by scar tissue inside the penis.

Physician assistant   Health professional who has a license to practice medicine under the supervision of a doctor. These professionals often are part of a team and may have much contact with patients.

Placebo   An inert sugar pill that produces a desired effect more by psychological suggestion than by physical action.

Plaque   Platelike accumulation of substances in the body. In the mouth, plaque is a sticky film on teeth that is formed by and contains bacteria. In arteries, plaque is an atherosclerotic lesion. In the brain, plaque is a lesion of tissue that is characteristic of Alzheimer's disease. Called senile plaque, it consists of a dense core composed mainly of beta-amyloid protein and is often surrounded by a cluster of degenerating axons.

Platelets   Small disks in the blood that assist in clotting.

Polyp   Small piece of bulging tissue. In the colon, a polyp may be benign or cancerous.

Prehypertension   Slightly elevated blood pressure that warns of possible future hypertension.

Presbycusis   High-frequency hearing loss.

Presbyopia   The inability to focus on near objects that results from loss of elasticity in the lenses of the eyes.

Primary care physician   Physician who coordinates patients' care, refers them to specialists, and provides all the medical care not requiring referral to specialists.

Prostaglandins   Naturally occurring fatty acids that have hormonelike actions, such as controlling blood pressure.

Prostate-specific antigen   Substance that increases in patients with prostate cancer.

Prostatic hyperplasia, benign   Enlargement of the prostate.

Prostatitis   Inflammation of the prostate gland.

Pruritis   Itching.

Psychotherapy   Treatment of a disorder by psychological means.

Public plan option   Health insurance coverage that would be managed by the federal or state government.

Radical mastectomy   Removal of the entire breast, some lymph nodes under the arm, and some chest muscle.

Radiologist   Physician who specializes in radiology, including X-rays, magnetic resonance imaging, and computed tomography scans.

Registered nurse   Nurse who has graduated from a nursing education program and is licensed by the state. Responsible for overseeing patient care and for educating patients and their families as necessary.

REM sleep   Rapid eye movement sleep; the least restful stage of sleep, in which there is more dreaming.

Renal   Referring to the kidneys.

Resorption   Breakdown and assimilation.

Restless legs syndrome   A condition causing people to feel sensations in their legs such as tingling, pins and needles, or crawling.

Retina   Nerve cells at the back of the eyeball that transmit information about light to the optic nerve.

Rheumatoid arthritis   An autoimmune type of arthritis that is much more severe than osteoarthritis.

Septicemia   An infection in the bloodstream.

Shingles   Painful skin rash caused by the chickenpox (herpes zoster) virus.

Sigmoidoscopy   An examination of the sigmoid (lower) colon and rectum.

Skilled nursing facility   Hospital-like nursing home.

Squamous cells   Cells in the middle layer of the epidermis; named for their scaly appearance.

Stent   A metal or plastic tube that is inserted into an anatomical vessel (such as an artery or a bile duct) to keep a previously closed passageway open.

Strangury   Straining to urinate.

Synapse   The connecting point between two neurons, where an impulse is passed from one neuron to the next.

Syncope   Fainting caused by too little oxygen reaching the brain.

Systolic blood pressure   The pressure exerted on blood vessel walls when the heart contracts; the higher number in the blood pressure ratio.

Thrombolysis   Breakdown of a blood clot.

Thrombus   Blood clot.

Tinnitus   Ringing or roaring in the ears unheard by anyone else.

Tympanum   Eardrum.

Vagus nerves   Nerves that lead to and from the medulla (a lower portion of the brain), connecting the brain with the heart and other internal organs.

Ventricles   Lower chambers of the heart.

Ventricular   Referring to the ventricles of the heart.

BIBLIOGRAPHY

Achenbaum, W. A. Morley's *A Brief History of Geriatrics. The Journals of Geron-tology* Series A: *Biological Sciences and Medical Sciences* 59: 1153, 2004.

Akpunoni, B. E., et al. Prevention of infective endocarditis: The new AHA guide-line and the elderly. *Geriatrics* 63: 12, August 2008.

American Cancer Society. Cancer. http://www.cancer.org/Cancer, accessed Octo-ber 10, 2010.

American Diabetes Association. Diabetes statistics. http://www.diabetes.org/dia betes-basics/diabetes-statistics/, accessed March 10, 2010.

American Geriatrics Society. http://www.americangeriatrics.org/about_us/who_ we_are/history/, accessed January 20, 2010.

American Geriatrics Society Foundation on Aging. Safe (and enjoyable!) sex for seniors: Tips from the American Geriatrics Society's Foundation on Aging. http://www.Healthinaging.org/public_education/safesex, accessed June 20, 2010.

Barker, W. H. Geriatrics in North America. In *Brocklehurst's Textbook of Geriatric Medicine and Gerontology,* 5th ed., edited by Raymond Tallis, Howard Fillit, and J. C. Brocklehurst, 1499–1509. Edinburgh: Churchill Livingston, 1998.

Barron, J. Brooke Astor's son is sentenced to prison. *New York Times* A31, De-cember 21, 2009.

Barry, L. C., et al. Higher burden of depression among older women. *Archives of General Psychiatry* 65(2):172–178, 2008.

Blow, F. C. Substance abuse among older Americans. In *Treatment Improvement Protocol, No. 26.* Washington, DC: Center for Substance Abuse Prevention, U.S. Department of Health and Human Services, 1998.

Butler, S. M. Medicare Part B Reform. A special report to the House Ways and Means Committee, No. 4, February 15, 1995.

Cassidy, E.L. Infantilization of the elderly in the institutional environment. *Electronic Doctoral Dissertations for UMass Amherst.* Paper AAI9737511, 1997. http://scholarworks.umass.edu/dissertations/AAI9737511.

Centers for Disease Control and Prevention. Prevention of pneumococcal disease: Recommendations of the Advisory Committee on Immunization Practices (ACIP). 1997. http://www.cdc.gov/mmwr/preview/mmwrhtml/00047135.htm, accessed April 13, 2010.

Centers for Disease Control and Prevention. Deaths: Final data for 2006. http://www.cdc.gov/nchs/FASTATS/deaths.htm, 2006, accessed September 25, 2009.

Centers for Disease Control and Prevention. National Center for Health Statistics. National Health Interview Survey. Celebrating the first 50 years: 1957–2007. http://www.cdc.gov/NCHS/NHIS.HTM, 2007, accessed May 28, 2008.

Chan, A.T., et al. Aspirin use and survival after diagnosis of colorectal cancer. *Journal of the American Medical Association* 302: 649–659, 2009.

Cousins, N. *Anatomy of an Illness as Perceived by the Patient: Reflections on Healing and Regeneration.* New York: Norton, 1979.

Cui, Y., et al. Body mass and stage of breast cancer at diagnosis. *International Journal of Cancer* 98: 279–283, 2002.

Czech, C., et al. Apolipoprotein E-4 gene dose in clinically diagnosed Alzheimer's disease: Prevalence, plasma, cholesterol levels and cerebrovascular change. *European Archives of Psychiatry and Clinical Neuroscience* 243: 291–292, 1994.

Di Bari, M., et al. Features of excessive alcohol drinking in older adults distinctively captured by behavioral and biological screening instruments: An epidemiological study. *Journal of Clinical Epidemiology:* 41–47, 2002.

Dieppe, P., and J. Tobias. Bone and joint aging. In *Brocklehurst's Textbook of Geriatric Medicine and Gerontology,* 5th ed., edited by Raymond Tallis, Howard Fillit, and J.C. Brocklehurst, 1131–1134. Edinburgh: Churchill Livingston, 1998.

Engelhardt, G.V., et al. Social Security and elderly living arrangements. *Journal of Human Resources* 40: 354–372, 2005.

Evans, J.G. Geriatric medicine: A brief history. *British Medical Journal* 315: 1075–1077, 1997.

Flatarone, M.A., et al. Exercise training and nutritional supplementation for physical frailty in very elderly people. *New England Journal of Medicine* 330: 1769–1775, 1994.

Flegal, K.M. Prevalence and trends in obesity among U.S. adults, 1999–2008. *Journal of the American Medical Association* 303: 235–241, 2010.

Gall, T.L., et al. The retirement adjustment process: Changes in the well-being of male retirees across time. *Journals of Gerontology Series B Psychological Sciences and Social Sciences* 52B(3):P110–P117, 1997.

Gibson, M.V. Evaluation and treatment of bone disease after fragility fracture. *Geriatrics* 63: 7, July 2008.

Glaucoma Research Foundation. Learn about glaucoma. http://www.glaucoma. org/learn/, 2010.

Goldbourt, U., et al. Paper presented at the American Stroke Association's International Stroke Conference, Chicago, 2010.

Grodstein, F., et al. Postmenopausal hormone therapy and stroke: Role of time since menopause and age at initiation of hormone therapy. *Archives of Internal Medicine* 168: 861, 2008.

Guimarães, K.C., et al. Effects of oropharyngeal exercises on patients with moderate obstructive sleep apnea syndrome. *American Journal of Respiratory and Critical Care Medicine* 179: 962–966, 2009.

Hoenig, M.R., et al. Early invasive versus conservative strategies for unstable angina and non-ST elevation myocardial infarction in the stent era. *Cochrane Database of Systematic Reviews* 3:CD004815, 2010.

Howell, T.H. Hippocrates on geriatrics. *Age and Ageing* 15: 312–313, 1986.

Howell, T.H. Avicenna and his regimen of old age. *Age and Ageing* 16: 58–59, 1987.

Hsu, J., et al. Medicare beneficiaries' knowledge of Part D prescription drug program benefits and responses to drug costs. *Journal of the American Medical Association* 299: 1929–1936, 2008.

Humphry, D. *Final Exit.* Eugene, OR: Hemlock Society, 1991.

Insurance Institute for Highway Safety. Q&As: Older people, http://www.iihs.org/ research/topics/older_people.html, April 2009.

John A. Hartford Foundation. A brief history of geriatrics. http://www.jhartfound. org/ar2005html/2_a_brief_history.html, accessed January 20, 2010.

Jones, D., and N. Bhattacharyya. Passive smoke exposure as a risk factor for airway complications during outpatient pediatric procedures. *Otolaryngology–Head and Neck Surgery* 134: 12–16, 2006.

Kaiser Family Foundation. http://www.kff.org/medicare/h08_7821.cfm, accessed September 30, 2009.

Kashner, T.M., et al. Outcomes and costs of two VA inpatient treatment programs for older alcoholic patients. *Hospital and Community Psychiatry* 43: 985–989, 1992.

Kübler-Ross, E., and D. Kessler. *On Grief and Grieving.* New York: Simon & Schuster, 2005.

Lehrer, S. *Explorers of the Body.* New York: Doubleday, 1979.

Levitan, R. Indian summer. In *Boulevards and Blind Alleys.* Albany, CA: Ruth Levitan, 2009.

Lindau, S.T., et al. A study of sexuality and health among older adults in the United States. *New England Journal of Medicine* 357(8):762–774, 2007.

Marrie, T.J. Community-acquired pneumonia in the elderly. *Clinical Infectious Diseases* 31: 1066–1078, 2000.

Martin, J.P. The elderly and surgery in the Middle Ages. *Vesalius* 14: 27–31, 2008.

Matthews, D.A. Dr. Marjory Warren and the origin of British geriatrics. *Journal of the American Geriatrics Society* 32: 253–258, 1984.

Mayo Clinic. Erectile dysfunction. http://www.mayoclinic.com/health/erectile-dysfunction, 2010a, accessed May 12, 2010.

Mayo Clinic. Urinary incontinence. www.mayoclinic.org/urinary-incontinence/types.html, 2010b, accessed April 18, 2010.

McWilliams, J.M. et al. Health of previously uninsured adults after acquiring Medicare coverage. *Journal of the American Medical Association* 298: 2886–2894, 2007.

Merck Manual of Geriatrics. http://www.merck.com/mkgr/mmg/sec7/ch52/ch52a.jsp, accessed April 13, 2010.

Miller, G. Do brain-training programs work? http://news.sciencemag.org/sciencenow/2010/04/do-brain-training-programs-work.html, April 20, 2010.

Moore, Senator Richard. Elderly driving statistics and motor vehicle operation laws. http://www.senatormoore.com/issues/indepth/seniors/resources/Elderly%20Drivers%20Research.pdf, accessed March 21, 2010.

Nanda, A. Hormonal therapy use for prostate cancer and mortality in men with coronary artery disease-induced congestive heart failure or myocardial infarction. *Journal of the American Medical Association* 302: 866–873, 2009.

Nascher, I. *Geriatrics.* Philadelphia: P. Blakiston's Sons, 1916.

National Cancer Institute. Breast cancer. www.cancer.gov/cancertopics/types/breast, 2007.National Cancer Institute. Colon cancer treatment. www.cancer.gov, 2009.

National Cancer Institute. Dictionary of cancer terms. http://www.cancer.gov/dictionary, 2011.

National Cancer Institute. Melanoma. http://www.cancer.gov/cancertopics/wyntk/melanoma, 2003.

National Cancer Institute. Study of tamoxifen and raloxifene (STAR) trial. http://www.cancer.gov/clinicaltrials/digestpage/STAR, accessed January 8, 2011.

National Institute of Mental Health. Older adults: depression and suicide facts (fact sheet). http://www.nimh.nih.gov/health/publications/older-adults-depression-and-suicide-facts-fact-sheet/index.shtml, accessed July 5, 2010.

National Institute of Neurological Disorders and Stroke. Stroke: Hope through research. http://www.ninds.nih.gov/disorders/stroke/detail_stroke.htm, 2010a, accessed January 17, 2010.

National Institute of Neurological Disorders and Stroke. What is Parkinson's disease? http://www.ninds.nih.gov/disorders/parkinsons_disease/parkinsons_disease.htm, 2010b, accessed March 22, 2010.

National Institutes of Health. Type 2 diabetes: Fact sheet. http://www.nih.gov/about/researchresultsforthepublic/Type2Diabetes.pdf, June 2008.

National Osteoporosis Foundation. About osteoporosis: What men need to know. http://www.nof.org/aboutosteoporosis/formen/whatmenneedtoknow, accessed January 5, 2011.

Obama, President Barack. The President's Proposal. Washington, DC: White House, February 22, 2010. http://www.whitehouse.gov/sites/default/files/summary-presidents-proposal.pdf, accessed June 11, 2010.

Olshansky, S.J., et al. Aging in America in the twenty-first century: Demographic forecasts from the MacArthur Foundation research network on an aging society. *Milbank Quarterly* 87: 842–862, 2009.

Poon, L.W., et al. *Handbook for Clinical Memory Assessment of Older Adults.* Washington, DC: American Psychological Association, 1986a.

Poon, W. The use of rating depression series in the elderly. In *Clinical Memory Assessment of Older Adults.* Washington, DC: American Psychological Association, 1986b.

Qato, D.M., et al. Use of prescription and over-the-counter medications and dietary supplements among older adults in the United States. *Journal of the American Medical Association* 300: 2867–2878, 2008.

Rabin, R.C. Benefits of mammogram under debate in Britain. *New York Times* D5, March 31, 2009.

Reynolds, M. "Little Boxes." Words and music by Malvina Reynolds. Oakland, CA: Schroeder Music Company, 1962

Ritchie, K., et al. The neuroprotective effects of caffeine: A prospective population study (The Three City Study). *Neurology* 69(6):536–545, 2007.

Sahyoun, N.R., et al. Trends in causes of death among the elderly. *Aging Trends, No. 1.* Hyattsville, MD: National Center for Health Statistics, 2001.

Scarmeas, N., et al. Mediterranean diet and AD (Alzheimer's disease) mortality. *Neurology* 69(11):1084–1093, 2007.

Schone, B.S., and R.M. Weinick. Health-related behaviors and the benefits of marriage for elderly persons. *Gerontologist* 38: 618–627, 1998.

Schröder, F.H., et al. Screening and prostate-cancer mortality in a randomized European study. *New England Journal of Medicine* 360: 1320–1328, 2009.

Seppa, N. A better test for prostate cancer. *Science News* March 14, 2009, p. 10.

Shakespeare, W. *Macbeth,* act II scene ii.

Social Security and Medicare Boards of Trustees. Status of the Social Security and Medicare programs. http://www.ssa.gov/OACT/TRSUM/index.html, accessed June 15, 2010.

Stefanick, Marcia L., et al. Effects of conjugated equine estrogens on breast cancer and mammography screening in postmenopausal women with hysterectomy. *Journal of the American Medical Association* 295: 1647–1657, 2006.

Stolberg, S.G. Obama urges Congress to avert Medicare pay cuts. *New York Times,* A25, June 12, 2010.

Thomas, D. Do not go gentle into that good night, in *The Poems of Dylan Thomas.* New York: New Directions, 1952.

Tinetti, M.E., et al. Risk factors for falls among elderly persons living in the community. *New England Journal of Medicine* 319: 1701–1707, 1988.

van Baarsen, B. Theories on coping with loss: The impact of social support and self-esteem on adjustment to emotional and social loneliness following a partner's death in later life. *Journal of Gerontology: Social Sciences* 57b: S33–S42, 2002.

Vickers, A. J., et al. Prostate specific antigen concentration at age 60 and death or metastasis from prostate cancer: Case-control study. *British Medical Journal* 341: 4521, 2010.

Warren, M. W. Care of chronic sick. A case for treating chronic sick in blocks in a general hospital. *British Medical Journal* 2(4329): 822–823, 1943.

Wiedemann, A., and I. Füsgen. Therapy for urinary incontinence in general practice. *Aktuelle Urologie* 40: 242–246, 2009.

Women's Heart Foundation. Heart attack symptoms: An action plan for women. http://www.womensheart.org/content/HeartAttack/heart_attack_symptoms_risks.asp, accessed March 18, 2010.

Woodson, K. The pharmacology of aging. In *Brocklehurst's Textbook of Geriatric Medicine and Gerontology,* 5th ed., edited by Raymond Tallis, Howard Fillit, and J. C. Brocklehurst, 169–178. Edinburgh: Churchill Livingston, 1998.

Yang, L., and K. H. Jacobsen. A systematic review of the association between breastfeeding and breast cancer. *Journal of Women's Health (Larchmont)* 17: 1635–1645, 2008.

Zoler, M. L. Marriage challenges change as couples become elderly. *Clinical Psychiatry News,* April 2008.

FOR FURTHER READING

Arab, L., and M. Sabbagh. Are certain lifestyle habits associated with lower Alzheimer's disease risk? *Journal of Alzheimer's Disease* February 2010.

Boden, W. E., and D. P. Taggart. Diabetes with coronary disease—A moving target amid evolving therapies? *New England Journal of Medicine* 360: 2570, 2009.

Chen, I. In a world of throwaways, making a dent in medical waste. *New York Times,* D1, July 6, 2010.

Dominici, F., et al. Fine particulate air pollution and hospital admissions for cardiovascular and respiratory diseases. *Journal of the American Medical Association* 295, March 2006.

Finkel, M. L. *Understanding the Mammography Controversy.* Westport, CT: Praeger, 2008.

O'Connell, H., et al. Alcohol use disorders in elderly people—Redefining an age old problem in old age. *British Medical Journal* 327: 664–667, 2003.

O'Connor, A. Heart attack symptoms differ according to sex. *New York Times* D5, March 31, 2009.

Sabbagh, M. *The Alzheimer's Answer.* Hoboken, NJ: John Wiley, 2008.

Sutter Health, http://www.sutterhealth.org/, 2005, accessed March 9, 2010.

INDEX

ABOUT THE AUTHOR

Carol Leth Stone has been a writer and editor of educational materials since the 1960s, specializing in biology and health topics. She earned a BA from Kalamazoo College, an MA from Governors State University, and a PhD from Stanford University. Stone's *The Basics of Biology* was published by Greenwood Press in 2004.